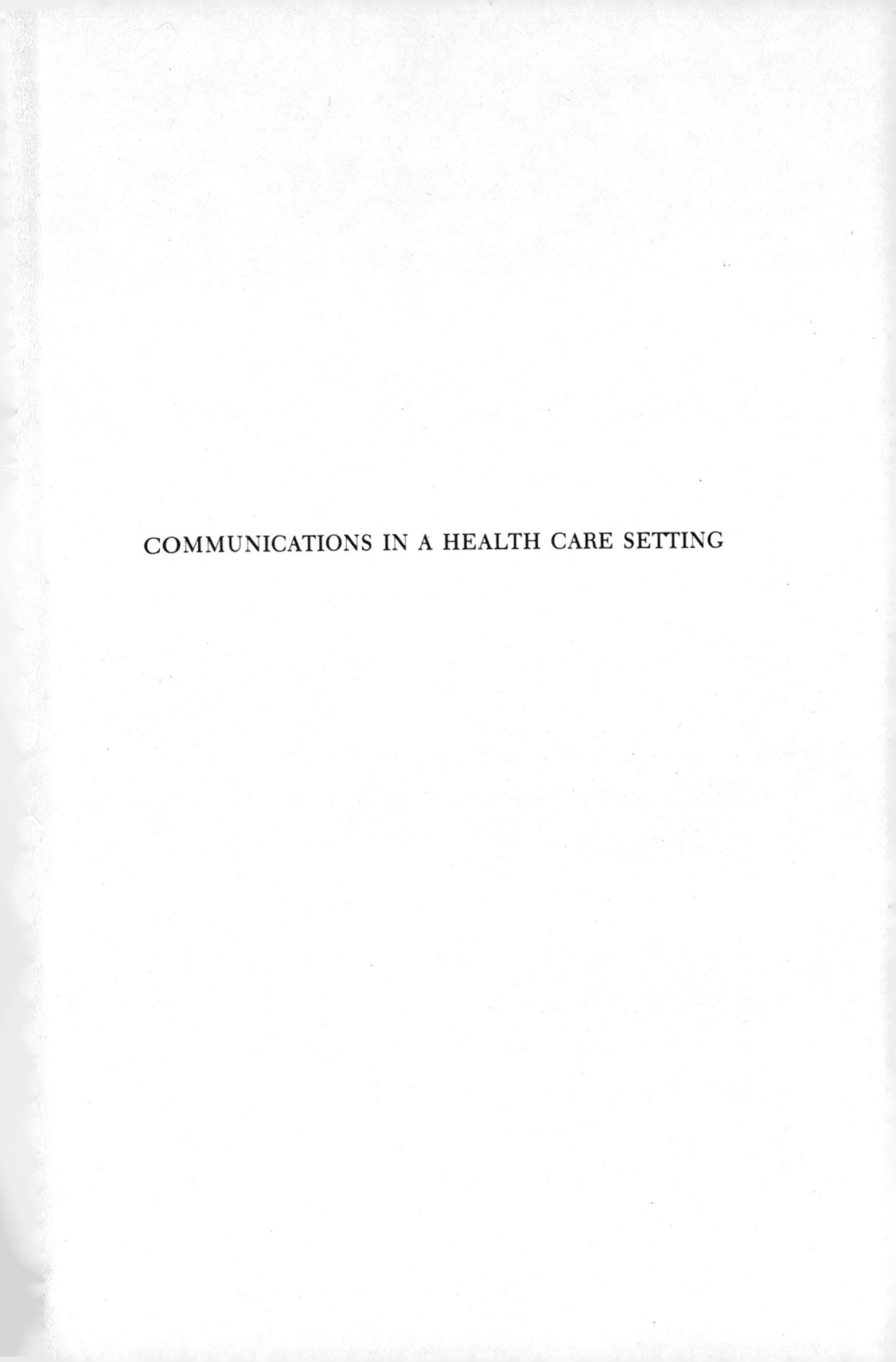

COMMUNICATIONS IN A HEALTH CARE SETTING

COMMUNICATIONS IN A HEALTH CARE SETTING

Edited by

MYRON G. EISENBERG, Ph.D.
Coordinator of Psychosocial Rehabilitation
Spinal Cord Injury Service
Veterans Administration Medical Center
Cleveland, Ohio

JUDITH FALCONER, Ph.D.
Psychology Service
Veterans Administration Medical Center
Cleveland, Ohio

and

LAFAYE C. SUTKIN, Ph.D.
Psychology Service
Veterans Administration Medical Center
Loma Linda, California

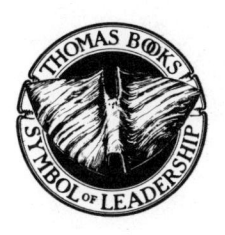

CHARLES C THOMAS • PUBLISHER
Springfield • Illinois • U.S.A.

W 84.1
.C 645
1978

Published and Distributed Throughout the World by
CHARLES C THOMAS • PUBLISHER
Bannerstone House
301-327 East Lawrence Avenue, Springfield, Illinois, U.S.A.

This book is protected by copyright. No part of it may be reproduced in any manner without written permission from the publisher.

© 1980, by CHARLES C THOMAS • PUBLISHER

ISBN 0-398-03963-1

Library of Congress Catalog Card Number: 79-17209

With THOMAS BOOKS careful attention is given to all details of manufacturing and design. It is the Publisher's desire to present books that are satisfactory as to their physical qualities and artistic possibilities and appropriate for their particular use. THOMAS BOOKS will be true to those laws of quality that assure a good name and good will.

Library of Congress Cataloging in Publication Data
Main entry under title:
Eisenberg, Falconer & Sutkin
Communications in a health care setting.

Based on presentations made at a conference held in 1978 under the joint sponsorship of the Veterans Administration Medical Center, Cleveland, Ohio, and the Paralyzed Veterans of America, Buckeye Chapter.
  Bibliography: p.
  Includes index.
  1. Communication in medicine—Congresses. 2. Medical personnel and patient—Congresses. 3. Interpersonal communication—Congresses. I. Eisenberg, Myron G. II. Falconer, Judith A. II. Sutkin, Lafaye C.
[DNLM: 1. Communication—Congresses. 2. Community health services—Congresses. 3. Delivery of health care—Congresses. W84.1 C734 1978]
R118.C62   610.69'6   70-17209
ISBN 0-398-03963-1

Printed in the United States of America
M-3

This text is dedicated to John Jacob DeJak, M.D., former Chief, Spinal Cord Injury Service, V.A. Medical Center, Cleveland, Ohio, whose unique communicative style has left an indelible mark on patients and staff associated with him throughout his many dedicated years of service.

CONTRIBUTORS

LOWELL F. BERNARD, M.S.P.H., Director, Cleveland Health Museum, and Instructor in Health Education, Department of Community Health, School of Medicine, Case Western Reserve University, Cleveland, Ohio. Mr. Bernard has served as a national consultant in community health education program development. He has appeared on local and national TV programs to discuss various aspects of health education and served as consultant to museums and health agencies in developing health education programs.

PATRICIA M. DEASY, M.A., M.S., Educational Liaison, Childhood Adaptation Project, a National Cancer Institution funded project, and Research Associate, San Diego State University, San Diego, California. Ms. Deasy's primary research interest is the investigation of how to enhance the quality of life for children diagnosed as having cancer, especially as it relates to academic performance.

MYRON G. EISENBERG, Ph.D. Coordinator of Psychosocial Rehabilitation, Spinal Cord Injury Service, Veterans Administration Medical Center, Cleveland, Ohio, and Clinical Assistant Professor, Department of Psychology, Case Western Reserve University. Dr. Eisenberg is active in numerous organizations concerned with the welfare of the disabled and received the Elkins Award from the National Rehabilitation Counseling Association in recognition of his work. He also received the first annual Olin E. Teague Award, presented by the Veterans Administration for outstanding contributions to the rehabilitation of war injured veterans. Dr. Eisenberg has published widely in the area of rehabilitation of the physically disabled. He is Consulting Editor for the *Journal of Sexuality and Disability* and Secretary of the American Psychological Associations's division of Rehabilitation Psychology.

JUDITH FALCONER, Ph.D., Psychology Service, Veterans Administration Medical Center, Cleveland, Ohio. Dr. Falconer works full-time with hemodialysis and renal transplant patients. She has also worked with the spinal cord injured and with physically and mentally handicapped children. Her research interests are in the area of communication skills development in hearing children of deaf parents.

NORA P. KERR, R.N., B.S.N., Coordinator, Utilization Review and Medical Audit, Huron Road Hospital, Cleveland, Ohio. Prior to this appointment, Mrs. Kerr held numerous nursing posts, including that of supervisor on the Spinal Cord Injury Service, Veterans Administration Medical Center, Cleveland, Ohio.

CHRISTINE O. MATHEWS, Ph.D., Director of Counseling Services, Student Development Center, Case Western Reserve University, Cleveland, Ohio. Dr. Mathews completed her internship and postdoctoral fellowship at the Cleveland Clinic Foundation, Cleveland, Ohio, where she evaluated and treated numerous chronic pain patients using behavioral approaches such as assertiveness training, biofeedback and operant conditioning.

MICHAEL G. McKEE, Ph.D. Department of Psychiatry, Cleveland Clinic Foundation, Cleveland, Ohio, and Lecturer, Department of Psychology, Case Western Reserve University. Dr. McKee holds offices in several professional organizations. He became aware of the pervasiveness of communications problems as an organizational consultant and family therapist.

MARY D. ROMANO, M.S.W., A.C.S.W., Supervisor, Social Service Department, Presbyterian Hospital, New York, New York. Mrs. Romano has practiced in acute and rehabilitation hospitals and served as a consultant to consumer and professional organizations concerned with the problems of the ill and physically disabled. She has published a number of articles relating to health care service delivery, the psychosocial aspects of illness, and management of staff problems.

Contributors

LYNNE C. RUSTAD, Ph.D., Medical-Surgical Psychologist, Veterans Administration Medical Center, Cleveland, Ohio, and Clinical Instructor, Department of Psychology, Case Western Reserve University. Dr. Rustad has worked extensively with spinal cord injury, renal and cardiology patients, providing consultation and staff liaison services on acute units as well as outpatient psychological services to patients and their families. She is currently involved in development of the CVAMC Cardiac Rehabilitation Program and research on psychological correlates of hypertension therapy. She has published in the areas of rehabilitation and sexuality and disability.

OLIVER SCHROEDER, Jr., J.D., Professor of Law, and Director of the Law-Medicine Center, Case Western Reserve University, Cleveland, Ohio. Mr. Schroeder's professional activities include service as a Fellow in the American Bar Foundation and membership on the Committee on Procedures on Hospitals and Discharge of the Mentally Disabled. Mr. Schroeder's expertise and interest in the area of forensic medicine and informed consent have resulted in numerous publications and lectures on these topics.

JOHN J. SPINETTA, Ph.D., Professor of Psychology, San Diego State University, San Diego, California. Dr. Spinetta is the Principal Investigator and Project Director of the Childhood Adaptation Project, a National Cancer Institution funded project studying children with cancer and their families. He has published widely and is recognized as a leading authority in the area of the psychology of the dying child.

CHARLES A. STENGER, Ph.D., Associate Director for Psychology, Mental Health and Behavioral Sciences Service, Department of Medicine and Surgery, Veterans Administration, Washington, D.C. Dr. Stenger, administrator of the world's largest psychology program, is regarded as the creative force behind the innovative delivery of psychological services within the VA health care system. Among his achievements was the development of programs to serve the needs of Viet Nam veterans and returning POW's and to sensitize VA personnel to these unique needs.

DENNIS G. STUART, Ph.D., Member, Core Faculty, California School of Professional Psychology, Fresno, California. Dr. Stuart served his internship on the Spinal Cord Injury Service at the Veterans Administration Hospital, Long Beach, California, and completed a postdoctoral fellowship in child and family psychology at Baylor College of Medicine, Houston, Texas. His research interests have included an examination of interpersonal climates on hospital wards.

LaFAYE C. SUTKIN, Ph.D., Psychologist, Veterans Administration Medical Center, Loma Linda, California. Dr. Sutkin's clinical and research interests are in the areas of medical-surgical psychology and assertiveness training.

ELIZABETH WALES, Ph.D., Associate Professor and Director of Medical Student Education, Department of Psychiatry, School of Medicine, Wright State University, Dayton, Ohio. Dr. Wales' widespread interests and numerous activities include consultation in medical settings and an extensive knowledge of patterns of nonverbal communication.

BARBARA E. YOCUM, M.S.Ed., Director of Counseling, Brookhaven College, Farmers Branch, Texas. Ms. Yocum's work in assertiveness training has included the design and presentation of numerous training programs in business, industrial, educational and medical settings for all levels of personnel.

PREFACE

Communications in a Health Care Setting grew out of presentations made at a conference held in 1978 under the joint sponsorship of the Veterans Administration Medical Center, Cleveland, Ohio, and the Paralyzed Veterans of America, Buckeye Chapter. Introductory comments made at this meeting are found in the Appendix.

Originally conceived of as providing continuing education to participants working in local, private, and public rehabilitation facilities, these annually convened conferences have gradually grown to the point where, today, they are national in scope. Each year the theme of the meeting has changed. The general issue of enhancing communication networks within health care settings was a problem often alluded to but not addressed directly at previously held meetings or, as it turned out, in the literature. A process that, in the words of one of our contributors, literally kills or cures the patient, has until very recently not commanded the investigative attention of the health care community.

The uniqueness of this text lies in its scope. Particularly significant is the inclusion of chapters on audiovisual techniques which can enhance communications, the medical record as an instrument through which one communicates, and the legal ramifications of the communications process. Certainly, there is an abundance of material produced which examines specific facets of communications not available, however, is a single text which draws together all aspects of the process and considers its role in the health care setting.

Practitioners must become knowledgeable as to the effect their communications, both verbal and nonverbal, can have on the rehabilitation process. Neglecting to do so can effectively undermine all effort previously or consequently expended to return to the community a fully functional individual. Failing to understand all elements of the communications process can be likened to the parable of the four blind men who, each feeling a different part of an elephant, surmised it to be something other than what it is. Such is also the case with communications: ignoring, for example, the importance of vocal intonation or facial cues can distort the verbal content of the message.

Communications in a Health Care Setting represents an attempt to cross disciplines and present varied theoretical orientations in explaining how the communications process works in the health care environment as well as provide suggestions as to how maladaptive communications patterns can be corrected. It is the editors' hope that through sharing this vital information with you, the reader, we will be able to critically reevaluate the impact of our interactions on patients and other staff persons and develop more effective and efficient interactional and informational communicative styles.

The editors' extend their thanks to Barbara Hampton for the care taken in typing this manuscript, and to Paul Cheremeta, National Vice-President, Paralyzed Veterans of America, Emmit Carmichael, President, and Luther Haskin, Service Office, Buckeye Chapter-PVA, whose material support have made the annual conferences upon which this and other texts are based a reality.

CONTENTS

Page

Preface... xi

Chapter

1. An Overview of the Communication Process in Health Care Settings. *Charles A. Stenger, Ph.D.* 3

Section I... 15

2. Mixed Messages and Missed Messages: Communications Gone Awry. *Michael G. McKee, Ph. D.* 17
3. Communication Problems and Perspectives: The Patients' Point of View. *Judith Falconer, Ph. D.* 35
4. Improving Physician-Patient Communication *Mary D. Romano, M.S.W* 58

Section II.. 69

5. Liabilities of Communication: Informed Consent—The Patients' and Professionals' Rights and Duties. *Oliver Schroeder, Jr., J.D.* 71
6. Assertive Behavior in Health Care Settings. *Barbara E. Yocum, M.S. Ed.* 81
7. Nonverbal Communication. *Elizabeth Wales, Ph. D.* 90
8. Communicating Within the Framework of the Medical Record: Need to Know versus Nice to Know. *Nora P. Kerr, R.N., B.S.N.* 107

9. Who Said Communication was Easy? Or Rebuilding the Titanic. *Lowell F. Bernard, M.S.P.H*...................... 112

Section III... 129

10. Facilitating Communications: An Aid to Effective Treatment on the Renal Dialysis Unit. *Lynne C. Rustad, Ph. D.* 131
11. Communications in a Health Care Setting: The Staff Perspective.
LaFaye C. Sutkin, Ph. D. 148
12. Coping with Childhood Cancer: Professional and Family Communication Patterns.
*John J. Spinetta, Ph.D., and
Patricia M. Deasy, M.A., M.S*................................. 173
13. The Role of Communications in Chronic Pain.
Christine O. Mathews, Ph. D. 206

Section IV.. 223

14. Spinal Cord Injured Patients' Perceptions of Ward Atmosphere Following Assertiveness Training of Nursing Staff.
LaFaye C. Sutkin, Ph. D. 225
15. Staff and Patient Perceptions of the Rehabilitation Process.
Dennis G. Stuart, Ph. D.. 243

Appendix
Opening Remarks, Sixth Annual Conference on The Care and Treatment of the Spinal Cord Injured. Paul M. Cheremeta, National Vice President, Paralyzed Veterans of America. 263

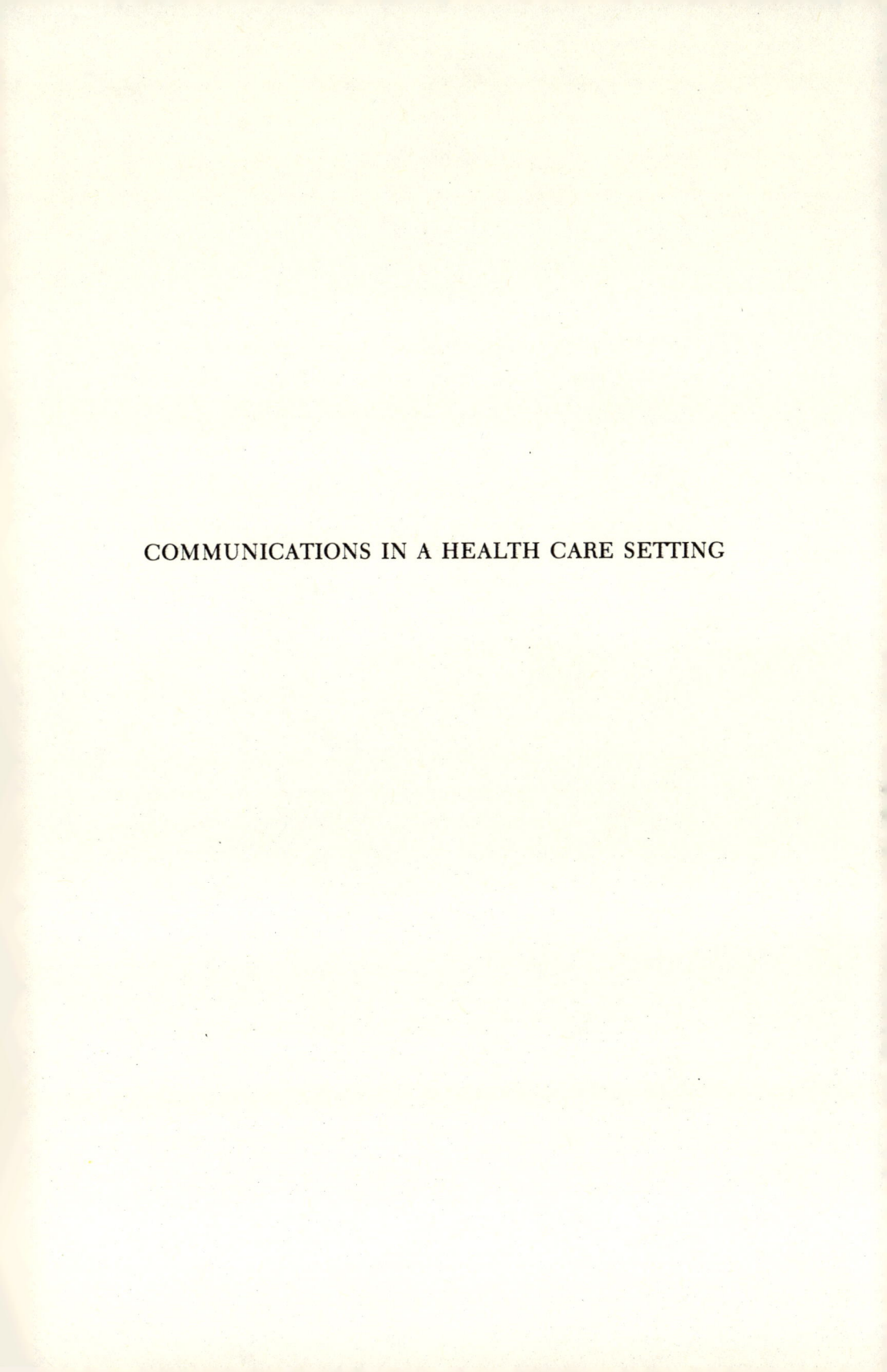

COMMUNICATIONS IN A HEALTH CARE SETTING

Chapter 1

AN OVERVIEW OF THE COMMUNICATION PROCESS IN HEALTH CARE SETTINGS

Charles A. Stenger

As a VA psychologist I became interested in communication processes about eight years ago when Vietnam veterans began coming to the Veterans Administration in large numbers. We in the VA system, many of whom were of the World War II generation, quickly communicated to Vietnam veterans that we did not like the way they dressed or acted simply because they did not look or talk the way we expected. At the same time they were communicating to us, "We don't buy that crap. If you're in a nice suit, you must have copped out to the establishment." The messages communicated were strong and the VA soon realized it had a major problem to solve. An effective way to understand and communicate with them had to be found in order to meet our responsibility of providing them services. We were created as an institution to serve the Vietnam veteran as well as other veterans and we could not do it if attitudes, theirs and ours, were negative.

To deal with this communication gap, a series of seminars were offered across the country where the leadership of the VA system met with Vietnam veterans and other young people. These confrontation-interaction groups proved to be stimulating and exciting. In the course of these meetings, an invocation was offered that embodies the essence of communication:

> Father, we know something about communication: joy and appreciation, pain and loneliness, tears, heartbreak, grief, gunshots, violence, wounds, blood, neglect, indifference, love, abandonment, sleep, death, no words. Eternal God, we cannot *not* communicate. You have not made us this way. Our prayer? He that has eyes, let him see the one next to him. He that has ears, let him hear the one next to him. He that needs us to go one mile, let us go two with him. Amen. (Braatan, 1971)

In this chapter, I will first discuss some good news and some bad news about communication and then attempt to identify some of the many ways in which we communicate. Next, I will discuss why communication in a health care environment is particularly powerful and important: It literally kills or cures patients. Finally, I will identify some approaches that might facilitate the communication process as a constructive force and that may be meaningful to patients and satisfying to you, the health care worker.

The good news is this: Everyone is good at communication. In fact, you are an expert at communicating. You communicate all the time and you are doing it this minute. This chapter is a form of communication. The way you receive it is a form of communication; the way you sit, read, and move around communicates to anyone around you, and to yourself, a lot about how you feel about it. You communicate whether awake or asleep, alone or with others, and *whether you want to or not*. The plain truth is there is no way to avoid communicating. Communication is as necessary as breathing, and we do it just as naturally. It is important to your survival to communicate effectively. Your personal satisfaction and the satisfaction of others is at stake.

Psychological testing and examination are based upon the fact that we are not only unable to avoid communicating but also that we cannot avoid communicating many things about ourselves. We sometimes think that we are able to present selected aspects of ourselves to others, but the truth of the matter is that in everything we do, in every communication process, we communicate how we feel about ourselves, how we perceive the world around us, how we view a situation, how we feel about sex, love, and affection. In everything we do, others (if trained to interpret) can perceive messages which communicate exactly what one's total feelings and perceptions of life are. Communication is a much more open process than most of us realize. We communicate everything.

I would like you to conduct a small experiment. Imagine a wall to be a piece of paper. Put a dot on that piece of paper. The way you placed the dot and the accompanying thought processes that occur provide answers to many basic questions about yourself. Those who said, "I'll put it in the center," probably went through this process: "I kind of want to put it in the center; I think I'll put it there." Others probably said, "No, I really don't want to put it there; I'll put it a little way away from the center." This may sound like a simple process but those of you who decided on placing the dot in the center of the page were really saying at that particular moment, "Keeping things in balance and under control are very important." Those who placed the dot away from the center of the page were responding to the same feelings but were saying to themselves: "I don't want to conform that much. I want to be an individual." If, however, a psychologist were to watch and ask what you were thinking when you placed the dot, you would begin to think about it much more consciously and quickly realize how much you communicate in the process.

So the good news is that you are an expert at communication. You may not see that as good news if you have discovered that you are revealing more than you intend.

The bad news is this: Although we are always communicating, we and others, do not always *hear* what is being communicated. How often have you been in a restaurant, sat down, been served, and then attempted to catch the waiter or waitress' attention for further service? The waiter or waitress sees around you, above, below and even right through you but does not see you. If you have ever been a patient in a hospital, it is likely that you have experienced similar feelings. The people around you do not really see, understand, or listen to what you are trying to communicate.

There is an abundance of good communicators but a serious shortage of good listeners. Most of us are poor listeners. Even if we attend to messages, we select out those parts we want to hear. That part of the message which we select to hear conforms to where we are at that moment—our beliefs, attitudes, and mood. If we are in the mood to be angry, we usually hear a communication that justifies our anger. So we are much better communicators than we realize and much worse listeners than we would like to believe. In part, we cannot be good listeners because we have trained ourselves to screen out those things we do not wish to hear. The following examples drawn from the health care environment support this statement.

Several years ago a study was conducted in which nine cadets from the Air Force Academy in Colorado Springs spent a weekend in a VA psychiatric hospital (Guyer, 1970). They were not there to observe patients; they were there to experience what it was like to *be* a patient. Air Cadets are bright, capable, and presumably stable and poised young men who are self-confident and competent to handle stressful situations. After two days in the psychiatric hospital, they all reported a reduction in self-confidence and their ability to cope with the environment. All felt isolated and lacking in human support. In general, all cadets experienced antitherapeutic reactions. Further, the cadets reported these reactions while describing the staff as being "good to patients." The psychiatric hospital was not an environment in which the cadets saw themselves as reflecting kind thoughts and benevolent attitudes. Within two days the impact of the treatment environment proved to be destructive. The cadets felt like psychiatric patients: They fell into states of apathy, dependence, and passive compliance. They reported experiencing anxiety that they might not be released after their brief experimental admission was over. Finally, they commented that staff appeared to be *completely unaware* of the devastating impact of the institutional environment and their role in that devaluing process.

A second example will serve to demonstrate the way in which this applies to all kinds of health care facilities—large, small, public, private, medical school-affiliated or not. Rosenhan (1973) reported a study in which pseudo-patients were admitted to a number of different facilities as schizophrenics. Immediately following admission, the pseudo-patients exhibited normal behaviors and attempted to communicate to staff that they did not really require hospitalization; that, in fact, they were healthy and should be discharged. Despite the fact that they had immediately resumed normal behavior, their length of hospitalization ranged from seven to fifty-two days. The consensus of opinions offered by these volunteers was that they simply ceased to be seen as individuals by staff. This loss of identity as individuals appeared to result directly from being labeled schizophrenic, but the same may have been true if the label given the subject had been paralyzed veteran, dialysis patient, etc. People tend to categorize, assigning labels to others. Categorizing patients reduces our sense of each as a unique individual thereby simplifying our interaction with that patient. The effects of labeling the volunteers in this study were to produce a feeling of depersonalization, a sense of powerlessness, and a lack of personal credibility. No credence would be given to anything they might say. They were tolerated in a friendly manner but never listened to or taken seriously.

The same is often done with patients with whom we work. As in the study involving Air Force cadets, Rosenhan found that staff were described as being composed of people who really cared. Yet, because the staff perceived these individuals as "patients," they lacked the sensitivity and awareness to treat them as individuals. In both of the above situations many crucial and accurate communications, including accurate communications from patients, were missed by staff members. They were unaware of the messages being communicated to patients such as, "You don't count as an individual, I care for you but I don't care about you," and other related messages. This data may be particularly significant because these studies were conducted in psychiatric hospitals, the purpose of which is to build people's confidence in themselves and others.

There are two related problems in the communication process that should be examined. First, we are not good listeners because we are only partially aware of the messages we give. Because we are unaware of all that we are communicating, we cannot recognize that to which others are responding. We focus only on our conscious messages. While the content of what we say may be what we consciously intend to communicate, it is possible our posture and other nonverbal cues are communicating a very different message to the listener. In any case, we often fail to fully recognize all that we are communicating. We pretend to ourselves that the words we are speaking are the real message, but the process is much more complicated than that. And, to the extent that we are not aware of the nuances of our communication, we are unable to understand why people respond as they do. It is unfortunate when we naively assume that the other person, the patient in this case, has responded only to our concrete message, failing to recognize everything else we have indicated by the tone of our voice, our stance, and our eye contact. If that is not clear, perhaps we should reflect on how convincing a waiter's question, "May I help you?" seems when viewed along with the other messages that had been communicated in the previous example. Most likely, we do not believe that there is any sincere interest when we have been ignored throughout our meal. The following anecdote may serve to illustrate how extraneous are the subtle communications that we give.

A man was sitting in his home watching a football game on TV. His neighbor, whose car was broken, dropped over and requested to borrow his car. The man replied, "No, I'm sorry. You can't borrow the car because I have to paint the upstairs room." It was clear that the man was going to remain watching the television for hours, so the neighbor looked a little puzzled, said "Thank you," and left. The wife, also looking puzzled, asked her husband why he had made such a ridiculous statement. He replied, "When you don't want to do something, any excuse is good enough." That is somewhat true. We only deceive ourselves when verbal communications are tempered with a pleasant tone while, in fact, we are communicating displeasure or refusal.

Because we communicate so much nonverbally, it is important to become aware of these other forms of communication in which we engage. It is possible that what we say or write is of little importance. Our tone of voice, facial expressions, and eye contact express far more accurately what we really mean. Think of all the common expressions used to describe these nonverbal components of communications: "His eyes narrow," "her eyes got wide," "his lips were a thin line." The color of your skin, and I am not referring to race in this case, communicates much more about your feelings than words can convey. For example, being "red with anger" or "pink with embarrassment" is a much stronger statement than saying, "I'm angry" or "I'm embarrassed." On the other hand, the natural color of an individual's skin (in this case, I do refer to race) is a basic part of that person's character and may communicate to another person, "You may like or trust me" or "We may not quite understand each other." If I am white, I may communicate symbolically just by my color that blacks better be careful; that they cannot trust me to care about or respect them. Similarly, our dress may give messages to other groups concerning many of our attitudes. The generation of the sixties denounced fancy clothes and opted for blue jeans. They were, by their dress, making the statement, "We don't buy complying with a society that requires too much conformity and distracts from individuality, so we're going to dress in a way that says we want to be different." Indeed, dress was a strong mode of communication, and older generations reacted strongly to that message. Hair was a particularly potent component of that message, one that spoke loudly enough to elicit physical aggression from others without the wearer uttering a single word.

Through our attitudes, overt and covert, we communicate much. Most of us are familiar with the existence of an abundant literature on body language. Body language, of course, refers to body movements, stance, gestures, etc., that communicate thoughts or feelings by how fast or how slow we respond. Similarly, we communicate by our presence or our absence. The fact that you are reading this chapter communicates that you have some interest in communications. We need also to remember that our communications are colored by things we have *previously* communicated.

Communication is a continuing process. It does not start at the moment we decide that we want to say something. It begins as soon as we are in the presence of another individual. We cannot turn communication off or on at will. We communicate by our appearance or our life-style. Such things can communicate that we do not accept society, that we are angry at it, or that we are different. By the time we speak, we have already communicated many things about ourselves.

Using all of the modalities of communications, we are continually communicating multiple messages, mixed messages, and confused messages. We usually cannot disguise that part of the message that indicates how we really feel about the other person. We may confuse the listener with content, but tend to communicate our attitudes toward them very well. Moreover, they tend to perceive whether or not we regard them with basic respect. We are usually much more "honest" in communicating how we feel about people than we intend to be.

Obviously, communication is vital in all areas of our environment, but it is particularly crucial in the health care environment. Why is this so? First, when we are ill and hospitalized, our world is more confining. We lack options to obtain reassurance or reinforcement as we might in other settings where alternative situations are readily available. The environment on a spinal cord injury ward or a psychiatric ward is the whole world for patients on those wards. The communications, the messages patients receive there, are what will sustain them. If those messages are unclear or not supportive, hospitalization can be a devastating experience.

I have engaged in an experiment occasionally that has enabled me to understand this more clearly. Visualize walking through the building in which you work, pretending that, in the course of walking through the entire building, you pass a number of people you know with no one acknowledging your presence. At the end of that imaginary walk, you have doubts concerning your importance and significance to others. If you have ever worked in a hospital, you know that it is very difficult for staff to speak to every patient they may pass in hospital corridors, simply because there are so many patients. As a result, an interesting phenomenon often occurs, particularly in psychiatric hospitals. As they approach a staff member, patients will usually look toward the wall or put their heads down. It is often easier to view this as a function of the patient's personality disturbance, particularly in psychiatric units when, perhaps, we should consider the possibility that they have learned that we do not acknowledge their presence. When we do not expect our presence to be acknowledged, it seems reasonable that we might take measures to minimize the discomfort, hurt, and unhappiness which results from being ignored. It is crucial to an individual's self-esteem to be recognized.

Because they do not have the opportunity to obtain feedback from other sources, patients depend on staff members to provide it. Visitors may be available intermittently, but they are not a part of the patient's basic existence. As a POW in World War II, I learned first hand the devastating effect of receiving messages that said I did not count and that no one cared whether I lived or died. These messages are blatant in a POW camp, but POW's had some reason to expect this behavior. If messages perceived by patients in health care and rehabilitation environments are not supportive, they are in big trouble.

The second reason why communication in a health care setting is so important is that the period of hospitalization is a particularly vulnerable phase of the patient's life. They are threatened by changes, physical or emotional, and experience fright, uncertainty, depression, and anger. They feel a lowered sense of self-esteem and an uncertainty about their ability to cope. They wonder what the future will hold. It is the very moment when positive reinforcement and stimulation are needed.

Perhaps because we have historically so poorly accepted the initiative for communications in the health care environment, the law now requires us to communicate. We are mandated to provide our patients the opportunity to give their informed consent to any procedure or treatment we might propose. Further, we are legally required to communicate certain facts, clearly and accurately, in the medical records of each patient so it may be available either to the patient or others who may care for him or her subsequently.

Given what we can see to be the importance of communications, it might appear that the simplest approach to resolve problems arising from it would be to communicate more frequently and openly with patients. However, it is not always easy for staff to respond to the demands and psychological pressure exerted by many patients desperate for reassurance. We get it from each patient; we get it from all patients. The demands on us are constant. How does one survive with the continuing demand for reassurance and recognition? What we tend to do is withdraw slightly. We become impersonal, protecting ourselves from feelings and the need to respond. We have made the mistake of assuming that if a demand message from the patient is heard, we must automatically submit to it. This is not necessarily true. The most basic message we can give the person is that they count enough for us to listen to and *hear* their messages. We can negotiate later as to whether we will carry it out, but we ought to at least acknowledge that we hear the communication. If not, we are saying that the patient is not valued by us sufficiently to command our momentary attention.

Practically, what can we do about these problems? The team concept is one practical way to protect a few members of the staff from being overwhelmed all the time. If one member of the team is assigned as the primary contact person and listener for a particular patient, the rest of the staff may relax their efforts with that patient. Individual staff members may then respond more intensively to fewer patients, thereby relieving some of the pressure. Using the team concept, patients can be helped to understand the situation from the start: one member of the staff will be their primary resource for information and communications. It can be simply explained that it is impossible for every staff member to respond to every patient so other staff members may not always be counted upon to respond fully. In such a situation, patients do not perceive subsequent inattention as a personal communication of their lack of worth.

Another problem commonly arises from the tendency we have to avoid being honest, open, and genuine with others. I believe we should try this approach much more frequently. The finest (and kindest) communication one can give to another person is one that demonstrates your willingness to be open and genuine with him even if you are conveying bad news. We somehow assume that if we cannot provide the desirable or pleasant answer, it will be destructive to answer at all. There have been a number of studies that have investigated the games that are played in the hospital with, for example, people dying of cancer. The staff plays out a charade. Everyone pretends that the patient is not dying. The patient is usually aware that he is probably dying; he suspects it but also engages in the game. Several investigators (Spinetta, 1974; Hersh, 1975; Goggin, 1976) have studied the phenomenon of children facing death. These studies suggest that even though staff thought it to be particularly important to protect children from the fact that they were facing death, the children felt cut off from their caretakers at the very time when they most needed relationships. We can communicate honestly even when people prefer not to hear the communication. They will respect our honesty and, more important, our willingness to be honest. Being honest requires having respect for the person. If we really respect somebody, we respect him enough to be honest and open enough to say, "I understand what you're asking me, but I can't do it, and here are the reasons why. . . ."

Another approach that can help us become more responsive and sensitive is participation in some form of sensitivity training or other type of interaction groups. Such an approach is an efficient means of learning to confront others, create understanding, and tolerate messages that we do not like to hear. Our deficits in these skills underlie many of our communication problems. If we do not wish to hear criticism, we avoid the person whom we believe might criticize us. The group process can be a useful tool in helping us build a tolerance for criticism.

Still another approach one can use to enhance the communications process arises from family systems theories (Ginott, 1969; Gordon, 1970; Patterson, 1971). One such concept suggests that ground rules unconsciously operate between family members which need to be identified. In family therapy, for example, an unwritten ground rule may be that father always speaks first. The order in which people speak is important, yet no one may ever have acknowledged that this particular ground rule existed, so that resentments which may have developed around the pattern cannot be dealt with. In any kind of communication process there are ground rules that each individual has developed, but of which each may be unaware despite the effect on the relationship.

There may be still one further obstacle to overcome in order to communicate effectively with patients. Often the information we have to communicate is of a highly technical nature and is most efficiently couched in a language with which we are very familiar but which may be "Greek" to the patient. In order to ensure the patient's understanding of difficult but important information, it is often most practical to rely on audiovisual aids. While the use of such materials is often thought to be so time-consuming as to be impractical, the reverse is more often true. The reduced time in repeated explanation usually more than compensates for the time it takes to initially provide clear and complete information.

Many other practical innovations and changes could be discussed that would help remedy existing communication problems. The most important step is taken, however, when we come to believe communicating effectively is worth the additional effort; that patients are worth the expenditure of energy as is the enjoyment we will derive from honest communication with another person. The experience of being genuine during the eight-hour workday cannot fail but to enrich our lives. Failure to communicate hurts not only patients; it hurts us. If we cannot communicate well with patients, most probably we are also not communicating well in other circumstances.

The movie, "Star Wars," contained the phrase "May the Force be with you." The Force is embodied in the communication process. It is being sensitive, sensing, caring, valuing, appreciating, recognizing, accepting, understanding and empathizing. Hopefully, in all our interactions with patients, the Force will indeed be with us.

REFERENCES

Braatan, R. Invocation. In *Viet-Nam Era Veteran: Challenge for Change.* Washington, D.C.: Veterans Administration Central Office, 1971.

Ginott, H. G. *Between Parent and Child:* New York: Macmillan Publishing Co., Inc., 1969.

Goggins, I. Psychological reaction of children with malignancy. *Journal of the American Academy of Child Psychiatry, 15,* 314-325, 1976.

Gordon, T. *Parent Effectiveness Training.* New York: Peter W. Wyden, Inc., 1970.

Guyer, E. G. Air Force cadets observe ward life. *Hospital and Community Psychiatry, 21,* 228-230, 1970.

Hersh, S. *Psychosocial management of leukemia in children and youth.* NIMH Report to Physicians No. 2 Washington, D.C.: Government Printing Office, 1975.

Patterson, G. R. *Families.* Champaign, Illinois: Research Press Co., 1971.

Rosenhan, D. L. On being sane in insane places. *Science, 179,* 250-258, 1973.

Spinetta, J. Personal space as a measure of the dying child's sense of isolation. *Journal of Consulting and Clinical Psychology, 42,* 751-756, 1974.

SECTION I

A broad spectrum analysis is an appropriate starting point for understanding communication processes and problems in health care settings. Each participant fills a specific role, be it patient, physician, family member, or other health care professional. It is within the confines of these roles that communication can become garbled, confused, or be missed entirely. That Alice in Wonderland is not alone in her communication problems is emphasized in this section.

Chapter 2

MIXED MESSAGES AND MISSED MESSAGES: COMMUNICATIONS GONE AWRY

Michael G. McKee

INTRODUCTION

Whenever people are together, communication is taking place. Communication has no opposite (Watzlawick, Beavin, & Jackson, 1967). It is impossible not to communicate to another person. Silence speaks as loudly as words, and inactivity as forcefully as activity. Verbal and nonverbal messages influence others who in turn cannot help but respond by themselves communicating.

Communication always takes place. It is *not* always effective. Communication goes awry for many reasons. The process can be amiss. If messages are given or received in a disturbed way, if they are not perceived at all, if they are badly timed and arrive too early or too late, or if they are inappropriate to the situation, disturbed communication results. Any element in the process can be disrupted in such a way that communication goes awry.

If there is distortion in the use of words, shared agreement on meaning disappears. Alice, in Wonderland, knows this well:

> 'I don't know what you mean by glory' Alice said.
> Humpty Dumpty smiled contemptuously. 'Of course you don't—till I tell you. I meant there's a nice knock-down-argument for you.'
> 'But glory doesn't mean a nice knock-down-argument,' Alice objected.
> 'When I use a word,' Humpty Dumpty said in a rather scornful tone, 'it

means just what I choose it to mean—neither more nor less.'
'The question is,' said Alice, 'whether you can make words mean so many different things.'
'The question is,' said Humpty Dumpty, 'which is to be master—that's all.'

This idiosyncratic use of words is of course not unique to Humpty Dumpty. "You're going to be okay," spoken by a health professional to a seriously injured person with permanent deficits may require as much translation of *okay* for the patient as *glory* did for Alice and may indicate more of a desire of the professional to be *master* of the communication than to be *accurate* in communication. "Don't worry about your sexual life" may make a spinal cord injured patient feel he's with Alice, in Wonderland, not in a hospital.

The communicator may also be disturbed, as in another example from Alice.

'She's all right now,' said The Red Queen. 'Do you know languages? What's the French for fiddle-dee-dee?'
'Fiddle-dee-dee is not English,' Alice replied gravely.
'Whoever said it was?' said The Red Queen.
Alice thought she saw a way out of the difficulty this time. 'If you tell me what language fiddle-dee-dee is I'll tell you the French for it,' she exclaimed triumphantly.
But The Red Queen drew herself up rather stiffly and said, 'Queens never make bargains.'

Some doctors never make bargains either. We're all prone to obfuscation and insisting on our own way, but the more power one has in a relationship, the easier it is to indulge these foibles. If doctors are threatened by straightforward communication, they can always be super scientific, telling the patient the truth in a form the patient can't understand. No bargain.

The receiver of messages, particularly if trying to cope with illness or injury, can also distort.

Coping behaviors in reaction to severe illness or injury include conscious as well as unconscious mechanisms. They are grouped into three main categories: coping mechanisms which are aimed at retreating and withdrawing from the threat, coping mechanisms that tend to block the threat or its significance from one's awareness, and coping mechanisms that serve to master the threat (Kiely, 1972; Verwoerdt, 1972).

Salient among those mechanisms aimed at withdrawal is regression, a movement back to earlier ways of relating to others, characterized by a narrowing of interests in the outside world, a self-centeredness, somatic preoccupation, and heightened dependency. Flexible withdrawal which is appropriate and conserves energy must be distinguished from surrender, a giving up which amounts to capitulation; in its extreme form it represents loss of "the will to live."

Other coping mechanisms have as their goal the blocking of the threat of death from awareness. In suppression there is a deliberate attempt to dismiss troublesome thoughts from the conscious mind. Denial can be targeted against the actual existence of illness, its significance, or the emotional aspects of the illness. In their milder forms, denial mechanisms probably help adjustment, but when denial is extreme and leads to neglect of medical advice, it is self-destructive. Rationalization may heighten trivial aspects of the illness, minimizing major ones. Depersonalization leads to the feeling that what is happening to one is like a dream, that it is not happening to one's self. Projection leads to blaming others for what is wrong, and this can be very difficult for helping personnel and families if they take the accusations and the anger personally rather than understanding them as coping mechanisms. Communication goes doubly awry when anger at one's fate, as a response to loss, is experienced by another as a personal attack. Helping personnel often find themselves reacting to anger in a patient by a mixture of guilt, defensiveness, self-righteousness, hurt, and anger of their own. The patient who is angry then gets, not empathy or understanding, but direct and indirect expression of bad feelings: abrupt treatment, angry words and looks, social isolation. Then the patient gets truly angry at the staff, and the basic issue of anger as a reaction to illness or injury is never joined.

Among those coping mechanisms which help to provide mastery and control, acceptance stands out; the loss is accepted, resulting in a loss of self-centeredness and a widening of interests.

The problem with inappropriate, badly-timed messages is illustrated in the old joke about the middle-aged man who felt the romance was going out of his marriage. His wife just didn't get a gleam in her eye anymore when he came home, he complained to his friend. The friend advised him to turn the clock back, to be romantic himself, to surprise her. So he ordered plane tickets to New York, got a babysitter for the weekend, went home Friday night and said to his wife: "C'mon—get packed—we're going to New York. Just like old times. We'll have a candlelight dinner, go to the theatre, a hotel room at the Ritz." His wife looked at him with a jaundiced eye, and said: "Well, if that isn't the last straw. The garbage men are on strike, the disposal breaks, Johnny gets sent home from school, the baby's sick, and you come home drunk!"

Correcting disturbed communication requires identifying the nature of the disturbances, their causes, and then effecting corrections, including abandoning inappropriate assumptions and distorted beliefs—not being Humpty Dumpty, The Red Queen, or the too surprising spouse.

OMISSIONS IN SENDING MESSAGES

The most common problem in sending messages to seriously injured people is probably that of not communicating full and accurate information about the injuries and what those injured can expect for themselves in the future (Cartwright, 1964). There are several studies which have shown that patients in general tend to be more dissatisfied about the information they receive from their physicians than they are about any other aspect of medical care (Waitzkin & Stoeckle, 1972). Contradictory, insufficient, or confusing messages are indicted repeatedly as the major culprits in hospital patients' unhappiness with their treatment. There is, however, very little research on why this problem exists, and that in itself may be one of the reasons why it does exist.

Reason for the Problem

Inadequate communication is an endemic problem in organizations. Consulting psychologists encounter complaints about communication in almost every organization they work with. In the sense that communication is the lifeblood of organizations, organizational anemia is universal, and those in this anemic environment find it hard to function in a mature, responsible way. Psychologically, important needs are served by being "in the know." The alternative, "being in the dark" is denigrating. Full communication with hospital patients is extra difficult because of special factors.

ADVICE WITHOUT DATA. There are many statements in the literature about how to communicate with ill people which have to do with what *ought* to be, what *should* be; these *should's* reflect the attitudes and beliefs of the writer but do not usually stem from observation and research on the communication process (Waitzkin & Stoeckle, 1972). Thus, physicians often have to rely on ideas such as expressed in a leading textbook of medicine which gives the following suggestions as to how a doctor should decide what to tell a patient:

> There should be no iron-clad, inflexible rule that the patient must be told everything. Few patients have the courage or faith or stoicism that the advocates of this conviction think they may or should have—how much the patient is told will depend on his religious convictions, the wishes of his family, the state of his affairs, and his own desires and character. But even this platitude solves nothing since it is not only the recognition of these factors, but the physician's wisdom in assessing the relative importance of each that determines how complete a discussion of the fact will best serve the interests of the patient. (Wintrobe, Thom, & Adams, 1970)

There is another set of opinions which seems to call for complete truth under all circumstances, regardless of patient's individual needs.

A third viewpoint, mainly applied to dying patients, demands distortion under all circumstances with the truth gilded, diminished, changed or omitted, presumably to preserve the optimism of the patient but possibly more concerned with the equanimity of the doctor.

This call to wisdom has been eloquently expressed: "to be a doctor, then, means much more than to dispense pills or to patch up torn flesh and shattered minds. To be a doctor is to be an intermediary between man and God. You must learn when and how to withhold truth from your patients if by not telling them all the facts of the case you can relieve or control them." This model honors authority and status, not honesty: "to your colleagues you have the obligation of civilized men sharing a great and noble task in fighting for a common cause of the great crusade. Medicine lives and is nourished by the great prestige it enjoys. Hence, never speak ill of a colleague, since to do so would be the same as speaking evil of medicine and therefore of your own selves" (Marti-Ibanez, 1960).

Exhortations such as these serve to guide physicians' behavior in confused and emotionally troubled waters.

And what do the data, as distinct from the personal desiderata, say?

What research there is on the subject indicates that the nearer the patient's desire for information is met the greater will be the compliance with instructions from physicians. The data also suggest that the more physicians' messages are mixed or missed, the more dissatisfied hospital patients will be with their medical care (Waitzkin & Stoeckle, 1972).

Spinal cord injury patients have much in common with chronic pain patients whose pain is not an accomplishment of illness or injury that is life shortening, and with psychiatric patients. All three groups have normal life expectancy but disorders that require monitoring by different health professionals. There often is initial hospitalization for months or longer, and anytime in the future there may be complications that require rehospitalization.

The emotional impact of the injury, pain, or psychological disorder is usually extensive; the patient having a sense of loss, feelings of inadequacy, devaluation, insecurity, and loss of control over his environment. Many new behaviors must be learned. For the spinal cord injured, this includes transferring to and from bed, manipulating the wheelchair effectively, pushing up regularly to prevent pressure sores, and getting in and out of the wheelchair, and in and out of an automobile. Social and verbal behaviors related to life in a wheelchair must also be acquired. For the pain patient, a "health role" with all its manifestations must replace the "sick role." The psychiatric patient must learn a wide range of coping skills so as not to be disabled by stress.

It has been observed that chronic pain patients provided with feedback information concerning their disorder (information which can include educational materials as well as internal cognitive and sensory information) are less likely to undergo severe stress and pain, especially when provided with informational material that they can self-regulate and can employ to estimate and avoid threatening aspects of their disability. In fact, the acquisition of a sense of personal control is *the* most important factor in rehabilitation of chronic pain patients (Gottlieb, 1976). Key cognitive factors such as learned helplessness, a sense of lacking control over stress events, an external locus of control, suppressed anger and related anxiety and tension expressed as cognitive-psychological events, are essential parts of the etiology and maintenance of the chronic pain experience, and by extension, of the "sick role" in general. Patients need information and knowledge to develop a sense of control, to develop skills within limits, and to feel valued and respected.

POWER. Caring for the patient's needs by using wisdom to define what information is appropriate to communicate may be the rationale for withholding information which is provided to physicians in their textbooks. Less honorable, but more human reasons may also influence the decision to withhold information. Power and fear are constructs frequently involved to explain failure to communicate openly. A physician's ability to preserve power in his or her relationship with the patient depends in part on ability to keep the patient uncertain, and on ability to provide cure (Waitzkin & Stoeckle, 1972). If cure is impossible, that fact may be suppressed because it would diminish power. And if uncertainty is resolved by admitting inability to cure, power would be twice lost. Thus, the forces work to preserve uncertainty by fogging communication.

FEAR. Seriously injured people may arouse fear in those treating them, fear that a similar fate may be lurking outside for the helper, or fear that relating empathetically may hurt deeply. Seriously injured people who will have continued, extensive handicaps are like the dying in this respect. Others may find it very hard to level with them because to do so is to develop a closer relationship that involves emotional grappling with the losses involved. Spinal cord injured patients who suffer multiple loss of function, and who do so often when they are young, are difficult for many doctors to communicate with. Identification with the patient can arouse powerful emotions that a physician may wish to avoid.

ENVIRONMENTAL CONTEXT. Studies of hospitals have identified

different "awareness contexts" in relation to patients who are dying. Some patients know they are dying. Some suspect. Some don't know. The combination of what each person in the situation knows about the other's identity and his identity in the other's eyes is the awareness context (Strauss, 1968).

An open awareness context exists when all know and acknowledge knowing to each other that the patient is dying. A closed context exists if the staff knows the patient is dying but the patient does not. A suspicion context exists if the staff knows the patient is dying but doesn't tell the patient, who nevertheless suspects the truth. A pretense context exists if the patient and staff both know the patient is dying, but neither admits to this knowledge.

The same range of awareness contexts characterizes communication with the seriously injured or ill patient, where the key data have to do not with incipient death but with the kind and degree of permanent dysfunction the patient can fairly anticipate.

Closed awareness and suspicion contexts exist in many hospitals. The professional rationalizations that would motivate closed awareness have been discussed; implementing the motivation is facilitated by the organizational system of most hospitals, one that is quite good at keeping truth from one patient, secreting medical records from the patient. However, suspicion often creeps in because the system is hard to make perfect: day and night staff give slightly different messages; some staff may work to sabotage the system, to ally themselves with the patient.

Impact on the Patient

While all the data indicate that many patients are not given full information about the true nature of the course of their recovery from injury or the progress of their disease, most interviews with patients and their families show that these people wish to receive truthful information (Waitzkin & Stoeckle, 1972). Without such information, one loses a sense of control over one's own life, is unable to make realistic decisions about compliance with medical advice, and is placed in a child-like role.

If a closed awareness persists for a dying patient, the patient is denied the opportunity to die with dignity. He can't face his grief, he can't talk to relatives about his impending fate, nor can he do the things one would do if death were imminent. In such a situation, the family and the hospital personnel are protected from many stressful scenes but they are also kept from what can be a satisfying participation in the rights of passage accompanying dying. Someone who is dying may be capable of an acceptance of death that the staff can share in only if there is openness of communication.

Spinal cord injury patients, who not only suffer multiple losses of function but who are subject to extreme emotional impact, with feelings of inadequacy, devaluation, and loss of control over one's body and one's environment, are likely to have all of those feelings intensified by a communication pattern which keeps them in the dark and treats them as incapable of processing full and accurate information.

SECOND PROBLEM: MIXED MESSAGES

Communication can be verbal or nonverbal. It can concern facts or feelings. It can be open or masked. It can be direct or indirect. Mixed messages frequently are characterized by a contrast between what is communicated verbally and what is communicated nonverbally. Verbal communication is often used to convey fact; cutting human thought, feeling, and action into slices like bologna; presenting simultaneous events in successive order. Gestures, expressions, inflections usually tell how one feels, whether one is happy, angry, sad, guilty, anxious, ashamed. Nonverbal communication can simply qualify the facts that are given, or it can contradict the facts, as in giving evidence that one is lying. One may express hope in words, despair in facial expression; one may express caring in words, indifference in action. Inflection may belie content.

Whether communication is open or masked, direct or indirect, determines whether a straightforward or a mixed message is given, and whether it is likely to be easily perceived or easily missed. If a doctor is angry at a patient for failing to follow instructions, an open, direct statement would be, "I'm angry that you didn't do as I asked." A masked, direct statement would be, "You'll have to keep this area around your bed more shipshape; this is a hospital." An open, indirect statement would be, "nurse, I'm angry that you don't get these patients working." An indirect, masked statement would be, "nurse, why are young men so self-centered?" That statement is masked in a common way, by being phrased as a question. Communication that is disguised or aimed at someone other than for whom intended is mixed and confusing. And it may be much more complex. Our culture may give us blinders that mask messages.

Henry (1972), in his remarkable book "Pathways to Madness," describes the complexity of emotional communication, and how anger is especially hard to communicate in its complexity:

> It is common among American parents, especially those with teenage daughters, perhaps, to experience an intolerable mixture of anger, fear, futility, desperation, doubt and self-righteousness when arguing with their children. Since the parent is often not sure of his own point, he feels in his anger he will never be able to convince his daughter; and since he no longer has the prerogative whether he is right or wrong, of beating her, he feels he can neither convince nor cow her. Hence, his growing sense of futility. Meanwhile, since he still believes that his daughter is in danger if he cannot protect her by dissuading her, and his own authority is in danger if he loses the argument, fear and desperation come to join his so-called anger. From the outside and to an untrained eye, the parent may merely seem angry: the emotions, however, are so mixed, or, as I have called them here, amalgamated, that it is really a question of whether the term anger should be used at all. What strikes us, then, is that to describe the feeling, the word anger is employed rather than the words "doubt," "futility," "fear," "desperation," "self-righteousness," etc.
>
> If Mr. Quigley is angry with his daughter Jane—with all the complexities of feeling this involves—often all that Jane, a creature of our culture, can perceive is that she is the target of anger, and she's usually unable to perceive the other emotions that are part of the angry display. As a creature of her culture, Jane is trained in blindness to the emotional accompaniments of anger; she therefore reacts to her father's anger as if it were merely that. These angry interchanges are often ambiguous interchanges not only because of lack of clarity in the arguments but because of this lack of training in emotional perception.

Impact on the Patient: Ignorance

To the extent that communication is indirect, aimed at an

inappropriate person, is masked and hard to perceive, the recipient may simply end up ignorant. This is a common status of hospital patients who feel devaluated and dehumanized, who feel uncertain and anxious. Mixed, in this case, means missed.

Contradiction

More complexly, patients are often given contradictory messages. While inevitably creating conflict, these messages at least give one choice. For example, a patient may be led by one health professional to believe there is hope for recovery of a certain function but also told by someone else that there is no hope. The patient in this case has a choice to pick either one to believe, thus resolving the contradiction. One is right, the other wrong.

Paradox

More complicated than a contradiction is a paradox (Watzlawick et al., 1967). Paradoxical communications bankrupt choice, leaving one with no choice, but with a demand for response. Ignore what I say. Think about that. If you ignore it, you paid attention to it. If you pay attention to it, you failed to ignore it. Heads I win. Tails you lose. And what if I ask my secretary: "Type the word "mike" and type that right or you're fired." The word "mike" can be either a person's name or a piece of electronic equipment. Well—capital M or small m? Either way she's fired.

The classic example of paradoxical communication is the double bind (Watzlawick et al., 1967). In a double bind situation, one person is in a relationship that has life or death significance, physically or psychologically. That person is given a message which states something, which also states something about its own statement, with the two statements being mutually exclusive. For example, if the message is an order, it must be disobeyed to be obeyed. "Put your arms around me and you'll feel better," say the words. "If you put your arms around me, you'll regret it," say the eyes. In a final and important step, the last nail is driven into the coffin of communication by a prevention of the recipient of the message from either escaping the paradox or getting away, by commenting on it or by withdrawing. "If you dare ignore me or challenge me, you violate a basic commandment." Therefore even though the message is logically meaningless, one is faced with the pragmatism of reality. You must react but you cannot react appropriately. It's impossible. Thus, the person subject to the double bind is likely to feel guilty, to feel punished for even suggesting or insinuating that there is a discrepancy between what he does see and what he is told to see. This behavior, if it goes on for a long while, contributes to schizophrenic thinking. The mother who says to her child "I love you," while holding him or her in a tense and rejecting manner, but refusing to let the child go; the mother who punishes the child for questioning her love is communicating one message in words, communicating the opposite message in actions, and forbidding recognition of the discrepancy. The message has unmixable ingredients, yet one must mix them and eat. The food for thought is poisoned. "Yes, of course you're still physically attractive," says the nurse to the paralyzed patient, "but I couldn't love you" says her body. "Don't you want me to give you a hug?"

Universities abound in double binds, as do hospitals. The professor has his role defined as "teacher of students." Thus, one primary message is to "get close to the students." However, on the other hand, a subtle message which is not put into words but is expressed in actions is "don't get too close to the students, because if you do, it means you are not loyal to the administration." Punishment, denial of promotion, may occur if one obeys either command. And if you charge the administration with hypocrisy, you may be denied promotion as a troublemaker.

Physicians often have many of the same double pressures on them. One demand is to communicate openly and directly with their patients and treat them as human beings. Another demand is to be a scientific god. Again, subtle punishment may be the reaction to failing either demand or challenging the incompatibility. The bind may be passed on: nurses may be told by physicians, "take care of the emotional needs of the patient but don't involve me." This may make it possible for the physician to give a distorted message to the patient which enables the doctor to leave the situation quickly, without questions coming up and emotions being aroused. "How bad am I." "You've got damage at C-3; nurse, fill him in afterwards," and unspoken—"but don't let him get upset." If the nurse does as the physician says in words, she will be contradicting the nonverbal message which is to support the physician in his posture and not produce upset. If she does not do as she is told in words, she is to blame for the patient's complaints about being kept in the dark. Whether the patient complains about ignorance or is emotionally upset with the truth, the nurse is at fault, yet she cannot accuse the physician of putting her in this spot or she is insubordinate. However, she has to do something. She cannot leave the situation. She has to act upon paradox.

This kind of double bind is inevitably passed on, in a case of the university, to the student, in a case of the hospital, to the patient. As a result, each becomes a pawn in a system that is dehumanizing.

At the extreme, the patient must deceive himself about his or her own internal state in order to support the doctor in the deception. Other responses are characterized by an obsession with trying to find cues that will enable one to solve the paradox. There is a shift away from the real issues in the situation towards searching for clues in the environment. One is hypervigilant. Yet since there is no key, it cannot be found, so the patient might simply give up and respond in a very concrete manner, withdrawing from emotional involvement.

Rehabilitation settings in hospitals may have in part a built-in double bind similar to that of a "therapeutic milieu" in the psychiatric community. In this setting, there are often antitherapeutic double messages to patients. On the one hand, patients are given the impression that they are adults who are responsible for their own lives. On the other hand, they are given to understand that their actions are beyond their control. The typical patient is supposed to submit to powerful authority in the medical community, but the rehabilitation model requires active participation in one's own care. One is placed in a child-like role and asked to act as an adult. A united front must be presented to patients at all times. As one writer states:

> ... the traditional relationship of the doctor towards the rest of the hospital staff makes difficult the freedom of communication and empathy that is requisite for a therapeutic community. For example, a departure by nurses from the nurse-physician relationship to which they have been educated raises implicit and often ambivalent struggles for power; the very nature of the issues and the ambivalence prevent much access to solution or even airing. In a traditional hospital ward, passivity, acceptance, and cooperation are the hallmarks of a good patient; efficiency, transmission of orders and messages, and sometimes kindness are expected of a good nurse; the doctor should know everything or at least be able to figure everything out. (Hoffman & Singer)

In a therapeutic milieu, in an ideal rehabilitation setting, the patient is asked to assume responsibility for much of his adjustment and progress. Yet, the pressure described above may transform the staff into united parental figures, communicating that they know the patients, their motives, and what is good for them, better than the patients do themselves. What can this produce but more and more childlike patient behavior and attitudes from those who are told in words to be adult?

In the amalgam of a therapeutic community in the medical model of a hospital setting, the nurses and other nonphysician professional staff are faced with an impossible task. On the one hand, at staff meetings, at rounds, they are expected to listen attentively to expert diagnostic assessment of the physician. In psychiatric units, in spinal cord injury units, in terminal illness units, these assessments usually emphasize severe handicaps of the patients, and the unlikelihood of their recovering from them. On the other hand, the staff is to give hope. Thus, they should understand the diagnosis but not understand it. Another factor forcing the same discrepancy is that the system says the nurse must understand the diagnosis to benefit from case conference but by definition must be less knowledgeable than a first-year resident, even if she has been on the unit for years. This is a mixed message which becomes a paradox when nurses are not allowed to challenge or discuss it.

There is recognition that physicians must change if the system is to change. Barber (1976) states:

> Patients are asking for more openness, more communication and more mutuality in these interactions, not simply to be treated (or managed) in a

better way, but to be part of a social system in which they have rights and even obligations that they have not had in the past. . . . The old system tells you not to talk with your peers or your patients and leaves all the decisions to you. The new system tells you to participate in a moral community in which there is discussion and communication with your peers, patients and other associates—welfare workers, nurses, paramedical personnel and so on. I think that the system is changing and that if physicians do not participate with interest and creativity, the system will change badly.

Note even here, patients and associates are not peers.

Even the call to mutuality is nonmutual. Patients increasingly are told of "patients rights"; they and their doctors are told to picture "managing partner" engraved on the patient's forehead. This is intended to emphasize that the patient is in charge of his or her own health care. But who in fact has the power in the relationship? Is there anyone who doubts the doctor is in charge? Back to Humpty Dumpty.

Negative Reinforcement

This kind of paradoxical communication may also constitute negative reinforcement for a patient in a rehabilitation program. Almost all communication has reinforcing value, either of a positive or negative sort. As the patient's role is confused, the messages are mixed, the impact is probably negative and retards one's own rehabilitative efforts (Fordyce, 1976). The messages are punishment.

There are also consequences in terms of feeling. Patients, nurses, therapists all feel dehumanized and alienated when communication is mixed. They are working together as a team to help restore functioning as much as possible and to enable dignified life given the disabilities that do exist. Their ability to do so is impaired by paradox. Feelings of anger, despair, and frustration are intensified. One feels literally in a bind. Paradoxes are stressful. One tenses thinking about them. "Don't believe me. I always lie." Someone who says that to you leaves you feeling stressed. Depending on how you react to stressors, your muscles may tighten, your breathing quicken, your palms sweat—you may have the whole range of physiologic reactions that make up the "fight or flight" reflex. And if the paradoxes persist, the reactivity persists, with subsequent debilitating psychophysiologic reactions.

RESOLUTION OF MISSED AND MIXED MESSAGES

This paper is addressed to problems, not solutions. But solutions do exist. First, the system may have to change. For the organization communication patterns to change, outside consultation will probably be required, since many studies of organizational change suggest that outside as well as inside pressure is required for change to take place. Second, the individual must communicate in a "CAREing" manner, with CARE being an acronym which stands for Communicate Authentically, with Regard, and with Empathy (Rogers, 1951). If skills are lacking or attitudes inappropriate, training is available.

Receiving Messages: (Missing and Catching)

Since sending is receiving and receiving is sending, the subject by definition has been covered. Some additional comments:

In receiving messages, some of the main mistakes can be summarized briefly as the 12 Ds (Don'ts) of communicating. If you want to miss a message, use a "D" or two. If a patient, for example, says "I don't want to go through that exercise today, I'm too tired," you can use these patronizing responses, these parenting responses.
(1) Demand: You will do that
(2) Deny: You're not too tired
(3) Deflect: Tell me what you're going to do later in the day.
(4) Distort: You mean you're uncooperative.
(5) Defer: I'll have to ask the nurse . . . doctor.
(6) Derogate: Tired, you just don't have the gumption to do it.
(7) Disagree: You couldn't be tired, you've hardly worked today.
(8) Diagnose: You're tired because you're afraid your wife won't visit tonight.
(9) Distract: Now let me tell you a joke. It'll cheer you up.

(10) Discount: Being tired doesn't matter.
(11) Debrief: What did you do to tire yourself out?
(12) Deprive: If you're too tired for this, you're too tired for the entertainment tonight.

Those don'ts can all be corrected very simply. St. Francis points the way:

> Grant that I may not:
> So much seek to be justified,
> as to console;
> to be obeyed,
> as to understand;
> to be honored,
> as to love. . .
> for it is in giving ourselves
> that we heal,
> it is in listening
> that we comfort. . .

The don'ts can be corrected by listening (Strauss, 1968). By active listening. By listening with one's ears as well as with one's eyes. By caring. Just as communicating and sending messages can be corrected by communicating authentically, with regard and with empathy, so can receiving messages be done in the same way, with authenticity, regard and empathy. If one listens warmly and empathetically and actively, the "don'ts" will be corrected. When listening, rephrase, encourage expression of feelings, check understanding with questions, label feelings, label silences, empathize, express your empathy, and respond warmly and genuinely (Rogers, 1951).

The consequences of the don'ts are alienation, despair, loss of esteem, loneliness, frustration and anger. The consequences of active listening are increased self-regard, emotional closeness, and the hope that comes from being understood. If you're a good fielder, if you don't miss the messages, you'll be caring fully for your patients. When communications go awry, be a "Catcher in the Rye."

REFERENCES

Barber, B. Compassion in medicine: toward new definitions and new institutions. *New England Journal of Medicine,* 295(17), 939-943, 1976.

Cartwright, A. *Human Relations and Hospital Care.* London: Routledge and Kegan Paul, 1964.

Fordyce, W. *Behavioral Methods for Chronic Pain and Illness.* St. Louis: C.V. Mosby, Co., 1976.

Gottlieb, H. Psychologically-oriented treatment program for the chronic pain patient. Paper presented at the American Psychological Association Annual Convention, Washington, D.C., December 5, 1976.

Henry, J. *Pathways to Madness.* New York: Random House, Inc., 1972.

Hoffman, I., and Singer, P. The incompatibility of the medical model in the therapeutic community. Unpublished manuscript.

Kiely, W. Coping with severe illness. In Z. Lipowski (Ed.), *Advances in Psychosomatic Medicine: Psychosocial Aspects of Physical Illness.* Basel: S. Carger, 1972.

Marti-Ibanez, F. To be a doctor. *M.D., 4,* 13-14, 1960.

Rogers, C. *Client-Centered Therapy: Its Current Practice, Implications for Therapy.* Boston: Houghton-Mifflin, Co., 1951.

Strauss, A. Sociological views and contributions. In E. Norbeck, D. Price-Williams, and W. McCord (Eds.), *The Study of Personality in Interdisciplinary Appraisal.* New York: Holt, Rinehart & Winston, Inc., 1968.

Verwoerdt, A. Psychopathological responses to the stress of physical illness. In Z. Lipowski (Ed.), *Advances in Psychosomatic Medicine: Psychosocial Aspects of Physical Illness.* Basel: S. Carger, 1972.

Waitzkin, H., and Stoeckle, J. The communication of information about illness: Clinical, sociological, and methodological considerations. In Z. Lipowski (Ed.), *Advances in Psychosomatic Medicine: Psychosocial Aspects of Physical Illness.* Basel: S. Carger, 1972.

Watzlawick, T., Beavin, J., and Jackson, D. *Pragmatics of Human Communication: A Study of Interactional Patterns, Pathologies and Paradoxes.* New York: W. W. Norton and Co., Inc., 1967.

Wintrobe, M., Thom, G., and Adams, E. (Eds.). *Harrison: Principles of Internal Medicine.* New York: McGraw-Hill Book Company, 1970.

Chapter 3

COMMUNICATION PROBLEMS AND PERSPECTIVES: THE PATIENTS' POINT OF VIEW

Judith Falconer

Health care systems resemble the blind men's elephant: what is perceived depends upon perspective and previous experience. Through repeated communicative interactions, participants in health care systems modify their perspectives. In a health care setting, communication includes attitudes, physical environments, roles and behaviors, the full range of verbal and nonverbal, intentional and unintentional messages. What is communicated to and by those in the system depends upon what each participant needs from the system, gives to the system, and takes from the system.

For the researcher, health care systems offer opportunities to explore new clinical areas; for physicians, to practice specialized medicine; for nurses to provide care for acutely and chronically ill patients; for psychologists, to help people develop those coping skills which facilitate return to health or adjustment to disability; for patients, the specialized personnel, facilities and treatments which allow return to health. Because participants enter the system with unique learning histories, expectations, personalities and special skills, especially communication skills, all possible desirable outcomes cannot be achieved; compromise becomes essential. Effective compromise requires open, continuous and honest communication between health care professionals and patients. Effective communication requires a shared language, common goals and agreement upon basic roles and behaviors expected from each participant.

Until recently, the physicians' perspective dominated health care systems. Other team members, especially patients, were compliant, followed instructions and accepted physicians' decisions. Recent legislative and judicial decisions require health care professionals to make every attempt to fully involve patients in their care. Patients are increasingly aware that they are entitled to full information about their medical status, prognosis, proposed treatment, in full or in part. The "living will" allows patients to make decisions about terminal care under carefully specified conditions.

It is extremely difficult for the already overburdened physician, nurse, therapist, or psychologist to meet the new legal requirements of health care consumerism. What do patients want? What do they think they receive? How can patients be involved in their own care? What can professionals reasonably expect from patients? What is a patient? Answers to these questions require an understanding of the verbal and nonverbal communication processes that occur between patients and professionals.

In exploring communication processes in health care systems, it is useful to examine how decisions about patient care are made. Traditionally, health care professionals developed skills through formal lectures and hours, perhaps years, practicing under supervision. Volumes of literature were read as part of professional preparation and continuing education. Such traditional training devices, which rely so heavily upon formal and informal verbal and nonverbal communications, are less effective in understanding patients' needs and perspectives. Consequently, those who work in specialized medical environments have sometimes felt they could anticipate and meet patients' needs only by drawing upon professional and personal experience. Such experiential bases would never be used as the only preparation to perform surgery, administer medication, prescribe a therapy program, or conduct a personality evaluation. Why then do professionals rely so heavily on experiential factors in their attempts to understand patients?

If a professional in one specialty wants to find out more about another speciality, it is relatively easy to seek out appropriate literature. But there is a lack of literature written by patients for professionals. Some books written by patients have received rather wide acceptance among target audiences and their families, e.g. Rollins, 1976; Oberley & Oberley, 1975; Lund, 1974; patient organizations produce educational literature. But patient-produced literature is seldom taken seriously by professionals. Professionals customarily read their own professional literature to the exclusion of that of other professionals, much less that of patients.

Just as professionals don't read patients' literature, patients rarely read the professional's. Patients are provided with simplified versions of procedures, routines, and schedules; but they are not expected or encouraged to read professional literature. In fact, patients who read professional literature are viewed with suspicion and perhaps accused of denying or intellectualizing; they are expected to rely solely on the information provided by those professionals directly responsible for their care.

In the absence of shared written communication, which is at least potentially precise, communication between patients and professionals is primarily oral and nonverbal and, hence, extremely imprecise. Communication becomes that exchange of information, attitudes, and behaviors which occurs between a single patient and a single health care team. Professionals remain suspicious of patients who obtain second opinions or travel to other health care facilities for consultation and/or treatment.

The fact that the patients' rights and health care consumerism movements have so rapidly become strong indicates that something is amiss in the communication process. If patients felt their rights, needs, and perspectives were being honored, they would not resort to litigation to codify the rules of communication. The health care professional is under fire and is being forced to look at health care from the patient's point of view. To develop effective communication patterns, professionals need an awareness of what it means to become a patient; for it is within that meaning that patients send and receive communications.

BECOMING A PATIENT

No one chooses to become ill or disabled; the role of "patient" is always involuntary. Societies and subcultures have widely different ways of treating the ill and disabled; attitudes toward the sick role greatly influence which individuals will become patients and at what point in the disease/disability process they do so. By the time hospitilization is indicated, the individual may have experienced considerable pain and have been a part-time participant in the health care system. Before becoming a hospital inpatient, the individual usually has had some experience as an outpatient. However, when the move from outpatient to inpatient occurs, professionals' expectations change. The inpatient must learn new roles and develop different communication skills. Furthermore, the inpatient must interact with a wide range of health care professionals: nurses, physical and occupational therapists, technicians, social workers and psychologists.

When hospitalization is indicated, the specific facility chosen is heavily influenced by the patient's financial status: individuals without adequate resources or insurance are sent to public facilities. Being a "welfare" patient may have a significant impact upon the attitudes of both patient and professional; patients may feel devalued in their own eyes or may feel that professionals are communicating devaluation.

By the time the decision to hospitalize is made, presumptive diagnostic labels have been applied that affect the immediate hospital environment. Labels determine the ward and room to which patients are assigned. Certain labels e.g., contagious illnesses dictate assignment to private rooms. Some labels mandate admission to highly specialized and highly traumatic specialized hospital environments. The specific label may invoke terror or relief in a given patient.

Once individuals assume the "patient" role, a variety of behaviors and attitudes are expected of them. Patients are required to remove street clothes; an important aspect of their identity is no longer available. Patients then notice the narrow bed upon which they must sleep; waterbeds, king-sized mattresses, and satin sheets must be left at home. Personal possessions are limited: cigarettes, food, and alcohol are restricted; over-the-counter and prescription drugs are forbidden.

During the first few hours, hospital rules and regulations are detailed, including such things as visiting hours, food availability and restrictions, recreational opportunities, toilet facilities, and bed operation. Individual freedom is rapidly reduced. Many of the routines which staff members take for granted require substantial life style changes on the part of patients. For example, a patient who works evenings may find it difficult to alter sleep patterns and meal times; yet professionals rarely ask what shift a particular patient works. Probably it wouldn't change the provision of medical care.

When patients submit to detailed physical examinations, many portions of which are embarassing, they are expected to be rather passive. These examinations are repeated several times during the first few days by a variety of physicians and physicians-in-training. Patients are questioned in great detail about aspects of their lives which, under any other circumstances, are considered private and not subject to probing. Frequently patients may not understand what questions mean and even if they do understand, they lack appropriate vocabulary to respond accurately.

Within the first few days, multiple diagnostic tests will be performed, often requiring patients to miss meals, consume unpleasant medications, and experience considerable discomfort, if not actual pain. Tests are scheduled at the convenience of hospital personnel; patients are "on call" for the entire staff.

While hospitalized, patients cannot continue regular employment, which may result in severe financial problems, especially if the condition is chronic, if residual disability is expected, or if a long recuperative period is indicated. Some illnesses or disabilities require patients to seek new employment, to develop new vocational skills, or to prepare for early retirement. Since most adults have considerable psychological investment in their jobs, the interruption of their roles as workers, providers, and bill-payers is potentially devastating.

In addition to economic roles, patients arrive in hospitals as occupants of a number of other social roles, e.g. parents, children, students, consumers, lovers, friends. They are suddenly transformed into quadriplegics, gallbladders, strokes, or any of the multiple diagnostic categories which determine and facilitate treatment. Patients lose all other roles, or the roles are subordinated to the prepotent role of patient. Other major roles are limited to visiting hours.

Patients also arrive at hospitals with set personality and specific methods of coping with illness and disability (Moos & Tsu, 1977).

The health care learning history of each patient is unique. In any situation, the best predictor of behavior is behavior in similar situations in the past. Patients' best predictor of staff behavior is staff behavior during previous encounters with health care systems. Patients whose previous health care experiences were traumatic or degrading have very different expectations of their current hospitalizations than patients whose previous experiences were rewarding and satisfying.

While the above changes are occurring, while the patients' behaviors and choices are so restricted, a considerable amount of time may be needed to maintain psychological stability, to assimilate new information, and to restore the body to health. But privacy is rarely available in hospitals. Even in private rooms, medical staff enter at will; if visitors are present, they are asked to leave. With less than private accommodations, patients may not even be able to choose silence as their companion; roommates may be addicted to television or have a steady stream of visitors. Moaning and groaning from nearby patients make contemplation difficult; deaths in nearby beds make thinking impossible.

Becoming a patient is a difficult, stressful process. Professionals who have any doubt that it is difficult to assume the patient role need only remember that physicians frequently adapt very poorly to that role, even though they receive both special care and privileges unavailable to other patients.

Within health care systems the roles of the various professionals are clearly defined. Participants usually know what skills, behaviors, and attitudes to expect from doctors, nurses, and therapists. The undefined role is that of patient. Various professional codes of ethics provide role stability across medical conditions: the physician, for example, is expected to behave the same way toward a patient with coronary artery disease and one with a fractured leg. But the two patients will face very different expectations.

Recent medical advances have expanded the role of patients in the provision of medical care. Consider, for example, the field of hemodialysis. When hemodialysis first became available it was an experimental procedure with little known about the patient's role in the process (Levy, 1974); programs, regimens, and techniques were developed as needs arose. Twenty years layer hemodialysis is an accepted and widely-used lifesaving treatment. Patients are now allowed, even encouraged to dialyze at home. This requires the dialysis partner to, in effect, function as a health care professional. The stresses of home dialysis are known at this time. It is rather strange, however, that although physicians refuse to treat their own families because of overinvolvement and lack of objectivity, they have allowed spouses to dialyze their mates. Such an expanded patient role places new demands upon the ill and disabled. Patients are expected to learn new techniques and procedures, to develop new communication skills, and to accommodate to very stressful situations.

PSYCHOLOGICAL PROBLEMS OF PATIENTS

With the number of changes occurring when people become patients, psychological problems, difficulties in adjustment, are perhaps inevitable. Customarily such problems received the attention of mental health professionals only when severe enough to directly interfere with treatment. More recently, however, medical psychologists are being assigned to specific patient groups and have routine contacts with all individuals carrying a given diagnostic label. Such deployment of professional resources allows problems to be identified before becoming severe. It also allows a more complete understanding of the emotional states experienced by patients, even those whose adjustment appears, or in fact is, adequate. At the same time, however, routine coverage may cause patients to think someone feels they are crazy. Furthermore, patients rapidly become aware that psychologists are frequently consulted to improve compliance, i.e. make patients behave in ways requested by health care professionals. Nevertheless, if professionals understand the psychological states of patients, they are more able to communicate in ways that meet patients' needs; they are more able to understand the patients' perspective.

A vast literature is available detailing general reactions to disability (Shontz, 1975; Cobb, 1973; Garrett & Levine, 1973; Moos, 1977; Eisenberg, 1977). Psychological problems of specific disabilities have also been rather thoroughly reported in the literature (Goldenson, 1978; Wittkower & Warnes, 1977; Marinelli & Dell Orto, 1977). Only a brief review is necessary for this chapter.

Nearly all patients experience elevated levels of *anxiety*. The new vocabulary, routines, smells, and machines are mysterious and confusing. Patients strive to obtain information to reduce and master anxiety. They frequently make incorrect assumptions about overheard conversations among staff members. Much time is spent waiting for physicians to "deliver the verdict." The absence of accurate information, delivered at the appropriate time, in appropriate language, greatly raises patients' levels of anxiety. Physicians are frequently engaged in no-win games: if they spend a great deal of time with a particular patient, the verdict must be bad; if doctors are rarely seen, it must be because they don't want to deliver bad news.

Many patients will tap multiple sources in their frantic search for information. They talk to other patients to "get the scoop." They attempt to coerce nurses into providing information. They ask technicians about test results. They coerce family members into asking staff for additional information. They read whatever literature they can find in the popular press, usually focusing on that which provides hope and encouragement. *Reader's Digest* and the *National Enquirer* become the patient's medical encyclopedias. Ultimately, only information and time will significantly lower the patient's levels of anxiety. In the interim, heightened anxiety, with its accompanying tension and autonomic nervous system arousal, exacerbates symptons, leads to new illnesses and slows the healing process.

As would be expected, most patients experience *depression*. Major illnesses and disabilities force patients to confront their own mortality. Even patients who rely heavily upon denial to refute the seriousness of their illnesses must deal with the fact that fellow patients become critically ill and die. Enduring pain depresses even the strongest individual. Patients who know that permanent disability or disfigurement is inevitable must work through their depression before they accept such consequences. In some cases, patients must make quality of life decisions every day: is life worth living with this condition?

Strong feelings of *powerlessness* and *dependency* are frequent consequences of hospitalization. Depending upon degree of disability, patients may be dependent in the most primitive aspects of daily care. Bedpans, urinary drainage systems, and intravenous equipment do not instill feelings of self-confidence and independence. Patients cannot make plans for their daily activity. Should their personal preference at a given time differ from that of the professionals, everyone knows whose preference will prevail. If patients cannot make decisions that are meaningful, they must depend upon the professionals' judgment. They must assume the professional has their best interest in mind when decisions are being made.

Patients are powerless to change hospital policies, no matter how inconvenient, irrational, destructive or anti-therapeutic they may be for a particular individual. Even the most minor aspects of daily life are controlled. Patients are left with only tiny areas in which independence and power can be asserted. Consequently, patients are forced to take extremely strong positions on issues that appear to be minor.

Patients also experience feelings of *depersonalization* and *dehumanization*. Everyone laughs in the movies when the young doctor refers to his patient as "the gall bladder"; the laughter is the discomfort of the familiar situation. Health care professionals *do* depersonalize patients; hospitals *are* impersonal institutions. Yet there is no more personal possession than our own bodies, which should be treated as complete entities, with extreme dignity and utmost respect. Patients desperately want reassurance that physicians and other health care professionals respect them as complete human beings.

When patients read their medical charts, they are seldom surprised to discover that little social data is included. The entries read: "This is the second admission for this forty-eight year-old white male, admitted for congestive heart failure." Laboratory data, in great detail, follow. Almost the entire chart deals with the organ system or systems affected by the disease. Where is the patient? Hopefully still on his narrow bed, wearing hospital assigned pajamas, and "patiently" waiting for the professionals' decisions and care. He certainly is not in his medical chart, even in skeletal form.

Patients may experience overwhelming feelings of *vulnerability*.

Staff members are capable of inflicting injury, either by commission or omission. Harsh words from a nurse may devastate a patient. Toileting accidents, vomiting, or spilled trays may precipitate placating patient behaviors. Staff actions may be interpreted as deliberately punitive: if pain medication arrives late, a patient may attribute the delay to anger at an infiltrated intravenous needle. Minor complaints may be withheld so staff members will meet more serious demands at a later time. Patients may be afraid to report incidents where staff members have, in fact or fantasy, behaved punitively for fear further punishment may result. Patients feel particularly vulnerable during the late evening and early morning hours. Fewer hospital staff members are visible, visitors have gone home, other patients are asleep; a recurring nightmare is that very bad things may now happen. One of the bad things is being overwhelmed with anxiety, depression, and fear.

Patients may experience significant amounts of *guilt*, especially if they feel they could have prevented or lessened the severity of the illness or injury. Such guilt may be exacerbated by professionals who are perceived as blaming patients for their illnesses. Refusal of specific treatments or noncompliance with medical, dietary, or pharmacological regimens may help patients assert their independence, but also raises levels of guilt and feelings of vulnerability.

Because family members may be involved in guilt induction, it is not unusual for patients to tell spouses not to visit for several days. The extra stress of family-induced guilt may be too much at that particular point in the treatment/healing process.

Feelings of *alienation* and *isolation* are relatively common, especially among the terminally ill. Patients are set apart from the rest of society by being in the hospital. Specific diagnostic labels may cause family members and friends to avoid contact, to physically withdraw from former patterns of closeness. Patients are wrenched from important social roles; the "patient" role does not fulfill all psychological needs. Although patients' illnesses or disabilities are at the forefront of all interactions with health care professionals, they are expected to avoid dwelling upon their physical condition in the presence of visitors. Even staff members may withdraw psychological support from the terminally ill (Klagsburn, 1977; Hay & Oken, 1977).

Although health care professionals are usually aware of the various psychological states experienced by patients, that knowledge in and of itself, has not been sufficient to result in effective communication patterns. If it were, patients would not become so upset by routine communicative interactions, even well-intended communications in health care settings. Attention to specific communication problem areas may increase awareness of the pitfalls of health care communications.

NEGATIVELY PERCEIVED VERBAL MESSAGES

A number of verbal messages which pass from professionals to patients are perceived negatively by patients. Examining some of these statements from the patient's point of view may increase awareness of routing communicative interactions during the provision of health care.

"I KNOW HOW YOU FEEL." From the patients' point of view, no other individual knows exactly how they feel. Unless you have been quadriplegic, you cannot know how quadriplegia feels. Training programs in some psychiatric facilities encourage interns to be admitted as patients for a limited period of time so they can experience being a patient. Yet simulations are simulations; they are not reality. For professionals to assume their education has made them fully aware of patients' feelings is self-delusional and self-destructive. Patients prefer that professionals become students and allow patients to teach their perspective.

Professionals sometimes assume that because patients may be inarticulate, their communications are less scientific, less valid. But patients can tell professionals how they feel, need to tell how they feel and want to tell how they feel. Patients want professionals to listen, to understand and to learn from patients as well as from books and other professionals.

"YOU SHOULDN'T FEEL THAT WAY. Patients frequently report being told their feelings are wrong or they have mislabeled their feelings. Feelings cannot be wrong; they simply are what they are. Feelings may be helpful or destructive to the healing and adjustment processes, but they cannot be "shoulded" away. Whether patients should feel angry when they are kept waiting, depressed when they don't immediately feel better, or discouraged by bodily disfigurement is irrelevant. Patients do frequently honestly experience such emotional states and being told not to feel in those ways does not change the feeling. It simply closes the communication channel and prevents growing to new and more adaptive emotional states.

"You don't really want to die." In some areas of medical care techniques and facilities allow survival without immediate concern for quality of life. Hence the "living will" movement. In other areas the quality of life may be acceptable to some patients and unacceptable to other patients. Patients and their families must make the agonizing choice of life or death. Even in less heroic situations, each patient must decide if the remaining quality of life is sufficient. In the process of making the decision, patients may need to say they want to die. At the precise moment patients say "I want to die" they probably do. When the health professional denies the reality of the patient's current feelings, the patient's opportunity to have assistance in making the choice of life or death is eliminated; the door of the communication process is abruptly closed. The patient, left totally alone, may feel obligated to prove he truly wants to die by attempting suicide. Other patients may use the statement to force professionals to pay attention, to devote more time, to provide more information, to prove that caring is a reality or to propose alternative treatments.

"Don't worry, everything will be all right." Staff members attempt to reassure patients by telling them their worries are premature or unrealistic, that time will take care of significant problems. Being told not to worry is like being asked not to think of a purple rhinoceros. The more frequently patients are told not to worry, the more worried they become. Furthermore, such statements disavow the real feelings of patients and fail to honor the patients' perspective. Patients do worry that the final diagnosis will be a fatal condition, that they will never walk again, that people will pity them, that their sexual lives are over. Patients' concerns are increased when professionals close communication channels. When patients express concern over particular conditions, professionals have splendid opportunities to provide the information, support, and encouragement that will allow the patients to confront the reality of the situation so feared.

"THAT'S AGAINST THE RULES." Patients feel that professionals reify hospital rules, regulations, and policies, accepting them as if engraved on tablets of stone and miraculously sent from on high. From the patient's point of view, professionals are frequently blind followers, unquestioning in acceptance of the hospital environment. Patients have no vested interest in the existence and smooth functioning of the entire hospital; their concern is limited to their own care. Long-term hospital goals are relevant only to the extent that they directly influence the quality or quantity of care provided to that particular patient. Since patients need to find small areas in which they can assert their independence, mindless rules are likely targets. Patients are not deaf; they hear staff members arguing that specific rules are antitherapeutic. Yet when the patients confront staff about the same rules, staff defend the rules. It is more realistic and therapeutic for patients and staff to work together to change rules or to subvert them if better care would result.

For example, it is against the rule in most hospitals for patients to openly consume alcoholic beverages. The rule may be appropriate for the acutely ill but inappropriate for the young quadriplegic hospitalized for rehabilitation. Some facilities circumvent the rule by having a physician write "p.r.n." prescriptions for one or two bottles of beer per patient. It is a great way to increase fluid intake! And it allows patients to continue a small part of their social lives.

"YOU'RE NOT TRYING." As far as patients are concerned, rehabilitation goals are very personal objectives. Patients' goals may not match those of the staff or institution. If patients are unwilling to work toward staff goals, it may be because the goals are inappropriate, poorly presented, or premature. Rehabilitation programs are established for the fictional "average patient." Has any professional ever seen that much touted "average patient?" Patients don't consider themselves "average."

When professionals reject patients' goals, patients reject professionals' goals and are then accused of being uncooperative, of failing to try. There is no way patients can win unless they allow themselves to be co-opted, unless they sell out to the system.

Every professional can undoubtedly think of a number of similar statements that arouse patients' wrath, indignation, or depression. Patients want professionals to listen to their own statements from the patients' point of view. How would the statement make you feel? What is really being said? Is there another way to say it?

NEGATIVELY PERCEIVED NONVERBAL COMMUNICATIONS

Nonverbal communications are even more subject to negative perceptions by patients. The problem is that in the nonverbal sphere, professionals may not even know that communication has occurred, much less that the communication was negatively received by patients. Every gesture, every piece of furniture, even staff time communicates a great deal to patients.

FACILITIES. Patients are particularly vulnerable to devaluation by the hospital environment. Nonfunctioning call buttons, small physical therapy rooms, limited recreation facilities, inadequate parking for the handicapped, and architectural barriers suggest to patients that their needs, and hence their bodies, are not important. Patients become very angry when the shortages in their area of the hospital are not evident throughout the rest of the facility. The way in which resources are allocated convinces patients that they are either valued or being shunted aside, tolerated. If the dialysis unit is at the end of an unlit corridor, with extra equipment stored in the hall, and furniture torn and shabby, patients believe that professionals view them as torn and shabby, merely being stored for the time being until someone better comes along.

Minor aspects of a ward may communicate more to patients than the professionals realize. One group of spinal cord injured patients were greatly upset by expensive wallpaper installed as part of a general ward redecoration scheme. Staff members sincerely felt that the redecoration had made the ward much more attractive. But the patients felt that, had the wallpaper money been spent on extra physical therapists or adaptive equipment, rehabilitation time would be decreased. The wallpaper evoked strong negative feelings and, as far as the patients were concerned, represented the administration's devaluation of the cord injured.

FOOD. Nutrition practices are particularly vulnerable to negative interpretation by patients. "They wouldn't feed this slop to their dogs but it's OK for us patients. They think we're animals anyway." When hospitals provide meals, patients expect them to be attractive and appetizing and to arrive warm. Patients who are learning the restrictions of a renal or diabetic diet may give up entirely if they assume that the food they receive in the hospital is what they will eat the remainder of their lives. How many professionals who work with such patients have tried the diet? The dietician on our renal unit just barely lasted one week!

TIME. Utilization of staff and patient time can convey very negative messages. Health care systems have rigid pecking orders concerning the relative value of the time of each participant. Patients are low persons on the totem pole. They become justifiably irritated when sent for X-rays and forced to wait in the hall for an hour or more. Doctors don't wait, nurses don't wait, only patients have time to wait. Yet patients correctly argue that the facility would not exist if there were no patients.

Much of the patients' time is spent waiting: for meals, for routine care, for physicians, for visitors. Each wait, each procrastination by a staff member, has the potential to produce disruptive emotional states. Since patients are aware of the pecking order, the three-hour wait for the physician may produce little direct anger; instead, the anger is directed toward the nursing assistant who arrives ten minutes late.

Patients know that time can be used punitively by staff members. Requested pain medication can arrive in 5 minutes or 5 hours. More difficult patients soon find that the delay is proportional to their behavior toward staff members. Patients can be punished nonverbally; and they know it. The message comes across loud and clear.

A very interesting aspect of the time dimension is patients' reactions to the speed of responses. If staff members immediately respond to a patient's question, the patient may feel that the staff member hasn't really heard, that a stock answer is being given. If the same professional stands and looks thoughtful for a brief period, the patient may be convinced that he has really heard and that the answer has been individualized.

PERSONNEL. The manner in which staff members are assigned to specific units within a hospital may be negatively interpreted by patients. If only new graduates of nursing programs are assigned to a particular unit, and even those leave at the first available opportunity, patients suspect they are not valued. If patients repeatedly complain that a particular staff member is insensitive, uncaring, and punitive but reassignment does not result, patients know that their point of view does not count; the continued presence of that staff member becomes a constant irritant. No words need be said.

Unsophisticated patients may not understand that personnel, especially interns and residents, rotate through medical services. Their new doctor orders the same tests and asks the same questions as the old one. Patients frequently wonder if the tests are even reported, much less interpreted. Patients feel they are guinea pigs, being used for training purposes. Even when the patient knows the physician will rotate, feelings of desertion and lack of caring can arise when the rotation occurs.

The number of ways in which nonverbal communications can be interpreted as negative messages by patients is infinite. The hypersensitive patient may see devaluation, rejection, and indifference lurking behind every bedpan. Only when patients feel free to verbalize those behaviors, practices, and facilities that upset them can the incidence of negative nonverbal communications be reduced.

IMPROVING COMMUNICATION

If the professionals remain aware of the patient's perspective, it is possible to alleviate some communication problems and to prevent others from occurring. Communication, and hence health care, can be improved by attending to three separate facets of patient care: information, skill development, and environment.

INFORMATION. As stated earlier, much of patient's anxiety arises from lack of information or inaccurate information. Health care professionals are the only individuals who can fully educate patients. The busy physician may not be able to explain each procedure to each patient, but conscientious use of audiovisual aids and health educators can reduce the burden and improve communication.

Patients frequently report that the doctor explained everything but they simply could not remember even essential details. Consequently, when asked if they had any questions, they did not. It is extremely difficult to formulate questions in areas in which we have no expertise. Those patients whose doctors have briefly explained details of a procedure, left descriptive literature, and returned to field questions, are both more knowledgeable and more comfortable. Literature prepared at low reading levels allows even poorly educated or foreign speaking patients to understand what will be done to them. The cartoon literature used with children to explain the birth of a baby or a trip to the hospital can be adapted for use with adult patients. Most people have limited powers of concentration and attention while ill or disabled. When information is spaced and patients allowed to learn in privacy, they feel like integrated, intelligent members of the treatment team.

It is also possible for patients to prepare educational literature and materials. Eisenberg and Falconer (1978) helped patients prepare videotapes on specific areas of concern to the spinal cord injured. The patients who participated in the project appeared to gain a great deal from that experience. They formulated answers to specific questions: they placed their experience in perspective. Some of them became leaders on the ward. When allowed to prepare such materials, patients find that their ideas and perceptions are valuable to patients, families, and even to professionals. Preparing materials in one area of concern also allowed patients to consider how they would respond to questions in other areas of concern; the experience generalized.

The fact that patients obtain much of their health care information from other patients need not mean that what they have learned is suspect. Well-informed patients can be a real asset to professionals; they are living proof that the treatment and procedures are tolerable. Patient reports are often much more credible to fellow patients than the more careful analysis by a physician.

Lack of attention to semantics in communicating with patients can cause severe problems. Many words have a very different meaning (or no meaning at all) to patients and to professionals. Take, for example, "exploratory surgery." Usually such a procedure is undertaken only after several presumptive diagnoses have been made. The operation is not exploratory in the sense that the surgical team is going in to "noodle around." Yet patients frequently report that they feel they are being used as guinea pigs because they don't understand the terminology being used by the doctor: the words are known but the tune is unfamiliar.

Semantics can also cause severe depression in patients. A colleague was consulted for severe depression of sudden onset in a patient. The medical staff thought treatment was progressing well and, all of a sudden, the patient seemed to give up. The patient reported that the doctor had told him they could no longer drain fluid from his lungs by a chest tube. The patient assumed that the doctor was saying that the fluid would now continue to build up and he would die. The fact of the matter was that other treatment methods were more appropriate at that time but the patient had missed that part of the conversation. No hope had been held out.

Some newspapers have a column that attempts to develop the reader's vocabulary: "use a word three times and it's yours." Not in medical settings! Patients feel overwhelmed by the vocabulary they are expected to acquire. The speed with which the necessary vocabulary is acquired is dependent upon patient's understanding of underlying concepts. Patients cannot feel comfortable with words like echocardiogram, autonomic dysreflexia and metastases in short periods of time. Consider how long it takes professionals to acquire the same skill. Simply because patients use a specific word does not mean they understand what it means. If a patient can explain his illness to his wife in the presence of his physician, a check can be made on his understanding and misinformation corrected on the spot.

A critical factor in the information dimension is timing: information must be presented at both the appropriate pace and at the appropriate time. It is a waste of time to explain fistula placement, hemodialysis and renal diets to a uremic patient with a BUN of 150. But it is downright destructive to wait to present that same information until the patient has been dialyzed three times. Patients need to know what will be done to them before it is done.

Presentation of patient information is an ongoing communication process, stopped only by the patient's death. Everything that a patient knows about his particular disease is acquired through communication.

IMPROVING THE HOSPITAL ENVIRONMENT. Those who work in a hospital rapidly adjust to the minor quirks of the building. If the air conditioner frequently breaks down, professionals go home at night and cool off. When they return, they should not be surprised to find patients crankier than usual. If elevators are slow or difficult to operate, professionals take the stairs. But patients confined to wheelchairs have no options; they must wait for the elevator, even if it takes days to arrive. It is important that the hospital environment be as comfortable as possible within its functional limitations. Patients can do a great deal to educate professionals on the shortcomings of the facility and can make useful suggestions for improvement.

Recent legislation demanding accessibility in public buildings has created a new expert: the handicapped patient. Those who live in wheelchairs can point out each and every barrier in any setting in a brief period of time. Professionals can probably never develop the acute awareness of the patient regarding such limitations.

This point was vividly brought home to a group of professionals when spinal cord injured patients were invited to a staff meeting. The professionals had been encouraging patients to participate in a hospital-based college program but encountered considerable reluctance on the part of patients. Why? A number of reasons. The hospital library was spacious but a wheelchair could not pass the circulation desk to get to the books and reading areas. There was no quiet place to study. Audiotaped class lectures were not delivered to the ward much less to the appropriate patients. Professionals were completely unaware of these shortcomings and difficulties, which could be easily remedied. When patients do not participate in programs which, on the surface, appear appropriate, they usually have very valid reasons.

Hospital visiting hours need to be carefully examined by the professionals from the patient's point of view. The psychological support provided by family and friends is both qualitatively and quantitatively different from that provided by professionals. Present policies seem to ignore some very important social realities. In many families both parents work, frequently on opposite shifts so child care can be provided. Unless visiting hours are flexible, the husband or wife may be able to visit only on weekends.

Patients also point out that, while professionals expect family members to provide care after discharge, schedules are arranged so that most patient care is completed before visitors arrive. Family members of spinal cord injured patients, for example, may never witness bowel care being done, yet have to do it several times a week after the quadriplegic returns home. If family members see that the professional is comfortable in providing needed care, the relative may feel more comfortable in providing that care later on. Yet the patients' wishes must be honored. If patients want privacy while care is being provided, visitors can be asked to leave the room. The patient must make the decision.

The hospice movement, rapidly gaining popularity in this country, resulted from patient's concerns about terminal care. Where hospices are unavailable, it might be worthwhile to create them in the regular hospital setting. The terminally ill patient has the right to be cared for in ways that will make the process of dying most comfortable. Terminally ill patients have a great need for honest communication, for involvement in their own care, and for respect, each of which requires careful attention to the environment's communications.

Professionals' openness to patients' perceptions of the hospital environment is essential to good communication. Even if specific aspects of the environment cannot be changed in ways suggested by patients, at least patients will feel professionals are aware of the problems and sympathetic. Patients will feel encouraged to continue communicating.

DEVELOPING PATIENT COPING SKILLS. If professionals are aware of those areas in which the communication process is particularly ineffective, they can help patients develop those coping skills which improve communication. Frequently this is interpreted as "make the patient see things our way." but that is neither essential nor inevitable. Two specific skills can serve as examples.

Many of the communication problems that arise between patients and professionals are a direct result of patient's nonassertiveness. Patients behave either passively or aggressively and fail to achieve their goals. Programs for assertiveness training have been developed that can be adapted for specific patient groups (Alberti, 1977). Such training can provide patients with those communication skills that will allow them to have a greater impact on health care systems, both in and out of the hospital. Assertive behaviors on the part of patients can reduce anxiety, powerlessness, and feelings of vulnerability. Currently assertive behaviors are most frequently observed in high status medical professionals.

Patients can also benefit from specific training in deep muscle relaxation and systematic desensitization (Rimm & Masters, 1974). When patients learn to relax completely and methodically, they feel more comfortable in the stressful hospital environment. They may also heal faster and develop fewer side effects. Patients need to feel in control while hospitalized and the self-control of relaxation training is preferable to that of tranquilizers.

Some patient populations may need a number of new skills, especially illness-related behaviors. Psychiatric patients, for example, may spend a great deal of time learning social skills that have been lost or never developed. The healthy take such things as asking for a date or scheduling an appointment for granted. But patients whose bodies have recently been mutilated or disfigured may need to practice the most elementary social skills. Because some illness-related behaviors are unique, patient groups have developed that allow recovered patients to educate the newly-disabled.

There are undoubtedly a number of other behaviors and skills that patients can learn to improve their communication skills in health care settings. If patients feel that their point of view is valued by health care professionals, if patients are assertive and relaxed, they are more likely to ask for new alternatives to maladaptive behaviors.

CONCLUSION

Everything in the health care setting communicates something to patients. Because the patients' perspective is unique, what is communicated to patients may be vastly different from what is communicated to the professional. Only by standing in the patient's shoes can professionals learn that vital perspective which improves health care communication and health care in general. Patients can teach professionals a great deal about the provision of quality health care. And unless patients are fully involved in their own care, delivery of medical services becomes a one-way street. The health care package offered by professionals may be marked "return to sender."

If health care professionals want to reduce the incidence of patients turning to "quacks," subscribing to untried treatments, and avoiding medical care until it is too late, it is essential to listen to those patients who are currently participating in health care systems.

REFERENCES

Alberti, R. E. (Ed.). *Assertiveness: Innovations, Applications, Issues.* San Luis Obispo: Impact Pubs. Inc., 1977.

Cobb, A. B. (Ed.). *Medical and Psychological Aspects of Disability.* Springfield: Charles C Thomas, Publisher, 1975.

Eisenberg, M. G. *Psychological Aspects of Physical Disability: A Guide for the Health Care Educator.* New York: National League of Nursing, 1977.

Eisenberg, M. G., and Falconer, J. *The Patient's Point of View* (Videotape film series available through Paralyzed Veterans of America, Buckeye Chapter, Cleveland VA Medical Center, 10701 East Boulevard, Cleveland, Ohio 44106). Cleveland: Veterans Administration Medical Center, 1978.

Garrett, J., and Levine E. *Rehabilitation Practices with the Physically Disabled.* New York: Columbia University Press, 1973.

Goldenson, R. M. (Ed.). *Disability and Rehabilitation Handbook.* New York: McGraw-Hill Book Company, 1978.

Hay, D., and Oken, D. The psychological stress of intensive care unit nursing. In R. H. Moos (Ed.), *Coping with Physical Illness.* New York: Plenum Medical Book Co., 1977.

Klagsburn, S. C. Cancer, emotions and nurses. In R. H. Moos (Ed.), *Coping with Physical Illness.* New York: Plenum Medical Book Co., 1977.

Levy, N. B. (Ed.). *Living or Dying: Adaptation to Hemodialysis.* Springfield: Charles C Thomas, Publisher, 1974.

Lund, D. *Eric.* Philadelphia: J. B. Lippincott Co., 1974.

Marinelli, R. P., and Dell Orto, A. E. *The Psychological and Social Impact of Physical Disability.* New York: Springer Publishing Co., Inc., 1977.

Moos, R. H. (Ed.). *Coping with Physical Illness.* New York: Plenum Medical Book Co., 1977.

Moos, R. H., and Tsu, V. D. The crisis of physical illness: An overview. In R. H. Moos (Ed.), *Coping with Physical Illness*. New York: Plenum Medical Book Co., 1977.

Oberley, E. T., and Oberley, T. D. *Understanding Your New Life with Dialysis: A Patient Guide for Physical and Psychological Adjustment to Maintenance Dialysis*. Springfield: Charles C Thomas, Publisher, 1975.

Rimm, D. C., and Masters, J. C. *Behavior Therapy: Techniques and Empirical Findings*. New York: Academic Press, Inc., 1974.

Rollins, B. *First, You Cry*. Philadelphia: J. B. Lippincott Co., 1976.

Shontz, F. C. *The Psychological Aspects of Physical Illness and Disability*. New York: Macmillan Publishing Co., Inc., 1975.

Witkower, E. D., and Warnes, H. *Psychosomatic Medicine: Its Clinical Applications*. Hagerstown, Maryland: Harper & Row Pubs. Inc., 1977.

Chapter 4

IMPROVING PHYSICIAN-PATIENT COMMUNICATION

Mary D. Romano

"Take two aspirin and call me in the morning."

This bromide has come, for many consumers of health care services, to characterize doctor-patient communications. Implicit in it is a physician who does not really listen to the patient, who gives a stock response, who temporizes and postpones, who takes but does not give. It is illustrative of the worst in doctor-patient communication in that it is indicative of such a breakdown in reciprocity that it has become a joke.

It might be said that in physician-patient communication, the entire process is predicated upon a sufferer turning to an expert in healing with the goal of ending distress. Inherent in the communications associated with this process is a combination of balance and imbalance. The patient, for example, is expected to tell the physician everything about himself without the physician responding in kind; thus, when a patient describes a digestive problem to his doctor, he does not expect his doctor to respond by saying, "You think you've got problems? Why my diverticulitis had me in the hospital for six weeks last year, and . . . ". Similarly, the patient is expected to tell the doctor details about himself which might ordinarily be kept secret but which are revealed with the patient's tacit understanding of doctor-patient confidentiality. This verbal imbalance is, however, mitigated by an assumption of reciprocity; information in exchange for alleviation of illness. Part of the process of alleviation extends beyond what the physician does, be it surgery, bracing, medicating, or whatever, to what the physician says, nonverbally as well as verbally, to the patient.

It is the posit of this chapter that both patients and doctors can be taught how to communicate with one another in ways that enhance the effectiveness of their partnership. The intention herein is to consider both some of the specific areas involved in this communication and to put forth some techniques for improving the communicating that occurs between doctor and patient.

Unlike the social small talk of a cocktail party, physician-patient communication is goal oriented. While this may seem obvious, the inexperienced doctor or patient may lose sight of this reality, in so doing missing both the actual or manifest message (what is said) and the latent message (what is meant or felt). This suggests, then, that the first issue for improving communication lies in clarifying goals. The patient's overall goal is to feel better, but this big goal is made up of many smaller goals; among these, phrased as patient questions, are "what's wrong with me?," "is it serious?," "can you reassure me about myself?," "can you fix what's wrong and, if so, how?," and "will I die?" It is in exchange for the answers to these questions that the patient talks to the doctor, and it is the patient's expectation that, in order to answer these questions, the doctor will listen.

Listening by the doctor is a largely nonverbal intervention skill, one that is sometimes called *attending*. Attending includes looking at the patient, observing him, nodding the head to convey maintenance of attention, and perhaps saying "uh huh" in an encouraging way for the purpose of sustaining the patient's verbal flow. Typically, for the doctor, the listening process is triggered by a series of questions directed by the doctor to the patient. Intimately tied to the nonverbal part of listening are those interventions that serve to facilitate information-seeking. *Specifying* is one such technique, in which the physician asks "when," "how often," "what color," and so forth. *Repeating the patient's words* is another technique, where the physician does just that: "belching a lot," "you feel tired all the time," "a funny, itchy rash on your hands." *Summarizing*, still a third technique, may be employed periodically during the listening process or at the end of it; when the doctor summarizes, he verbalizes a précis in his own words of what the patient has said. All of these physician interventions convey to the patient that the doctor has listened and heard accurately the manifest content of what the patient has said.

Part of listening by the physician, however, must include listening with the so-called third ear in which the doctor hears not only manifest content but latent content. It is the integration of manifest and latent content coupled with the doctor's knowledge base that allows him to diagnose the patient's problem. In order to verify his subjective impression of latent content, the physician can employ several communications techniques designed to elicit patient feelings. *Responding to feelings*, in which the doctor says such things as "you sound angry" or "this has troubled you a lot," serves this purpose as does *universalization*, in which the physician verbally attributes a feeling to the patient that is shared by others in his situation.

From the physician's point of view, listening or attending and the other communication skills related to it may present certain problems above and beyond the difficulty of mastering their appropriate use. One problem is that listening is a highly time-consuming process, and most physicians indicate that, for them, time is a commodity more precious and rare than expertise. Unfortunately, there is no ready, realistic solution to this problem. While it is conceivable that scheduling fewer patients, delegating responsibilities, and other efficiency efforts might give a doctor more time to spend listening with those patients he has, it is also the doctor's reality that illness is to some degree inherently unpredictable so that all the scheduling and delegating in the world cannot prevent patient emergencies or the other aspects of medical practice that consume the physician's time and energies.

A second problem engendered for the physician in listening is that listening involves skills that are not genetically based but, rather, are learned. It has been traditional in the United States that medical education occurs in two places; the basic, theoretical work is learned in vitro in the laboratory, and the clinical aspect of the work is learned in vivo on patients under the guidance of a physician preceptor who serves as a role model for the trainee. Thus, if the student has as a role model a physician who listens skillfully, the student will himself learn listening skills, but if the preceptor is a poor listener or one who sees little value in listening skills, then the student physician will be reinforced by the preceptor for modeling negative attitudes or behaviors. There is, in medical education, a true paucity of course material relating to the physician-patient relationship or to issues. One medical school that does have a course dealing with the physician-patient relationship is Columbia University's College of Physicians and Surgeons; their course is given to first year, first semester medical students who meet in small groups with preceptors and resource personnel whose task it is to help students consider varying aspects of the physician-patient relationship and some of the issues faced by physicians therein. As a resource person for this course, it has been my experience that both specific communication skills and their appropriate employment in given situations are a perceived need of the students, a need repeatedly highlighted by the structure of the course. This need, at least at present, is met by preceptor modeling rather than by structured course content offered at a time in the education curriculum when the student physicians are about to engage in extensive patient contact, i.e. at a time when behavioral rehearsals and reinforcement of skill would be most immediate.

The physician's third problem with listening is that patients are often poor communicators themselves; this problem can make listening onerous if not impossible for the physician. It can be hypothesized that patient problems in talking with doctors could be classified as falling into specific categories. First among these are the effects of physician deification upon patient communication. The patient, as noted previously, comes to the medical expert in search of cure or alleviation of symptomatology; as medical knowledge, material, and technique become more complex and rarified, the medical practitioner's armamentarium of information and skill increases his distance from the ordinary layman, making him esoteric, and as a result, increasing the propensity to endow him with magical properties. Until relatively recent years, the physician could be seen by his patients not only as a doctor but as a member of the volunteer fire department, a bowler, an alderman at church, i.e. a mortal being just like the patient. Medical sophistication and specialization have done much to set the physician apart from his lay peers, and with distance have come the burdens of mystery and of unrealistic expectation. Perhaps the most immediate effect of patient deification of the doctor upon the physician-patient communication process is the common presumption by patients that doctors can read their minds. In the perception of the patient who deifies his doctor, the physician will know everything whether or not the patient articulates it; this belief absolves the patient from responsibility and places instead a formidable responsibility on the doctor who is faced with the need to do the patient's communicating as well as his own. This is a classic no-win situation in which physician frustration and withdrawal are not infrequent options.

A second set of patient communication problems are related to patient anxiety as a response to the stress of illness. There is no doubt that the illness of oneself or of a loved one is an inherently stressful experience, and anxiety is the organism's means of response to stress. It is well-known that anxiety can inhibit both physical and cognitive functioning. A person who has been mugged, for example, may be unable to describe or recognize the mugger to the police because his anxiety was such that visual and auditory perceptions were not registering during the critical event. The implication of this is that patient anxiety can impair the patient's ability to listen and hear, resulting in skewed or inappropriate patient responses to questioning, oververbalization by the patient, and so on. This can in turn establish the necessary conditions for cyclic doctor-patient misunderstanding, frustration, and general miscommunication.

Related to anxiety on occasion is the area of patient discursiveness in communication. The discursive patient cannot stop talking; he is unable to discriminate how much information is too much or how many words are too many, and the stimulus overload that he provides causes the doctor's receptors to shut down or short circuit. When asked, for example, if he has a family history of diabetes, the discursive patient will respond with details of his grandparents' emigration from Europe, their work, play, and eating habits, those of his parents and siblings, the attitudes with which he was raised about sweet foods, his current eating habits, and a host of other irrelevant details. Lost in these innumerable details he may or may not fail to mention that his father and sister are both insulin-controlled diabetics. The discursive patient may communicate in the way he does as a part of an unconscious hostile process, or he may have a characterological impairment in social judgment which interferes with his ability to see the inappropriateness of his responses, or he may be talking to drown out his anxiety, or he may have had no practice in dealing with physicians, or he may feel an acute sense of entitlement ("I'm paying for this, and I'm going to get my money's worth; this doctor is not going to rush me out of here."). It can, however, be difficult for the doctor to discriminate the etiology of the behavior or to intervene to set limits on the behavior itself.

Indeed, setting limits is just one aspect of the active part of doctor-patient communication. If communication is seen as a complex dance of verbal and nonverbal stimulus and response, speaking and listening, giving and taking, then it becomes clear that problems associated with listening are not the only problems in physician-patient communication that must be resolved.

The physician-patient relationship is one in which the patient experiences vulnerability, initially grounded in being unable to control body process to the extent that he is sick and in need of professional help, and secondarily in that he reveals himself through communication to the doctor. The patient is the supplicant in this relationship; in the terms of transactional analysis, he is one down, and the doctor is one up, or the patient is Child and the doctor Parent. This inherent inequity makes for doctor-patient difficulty in the communication process, where an adult-adult reciprocal model is one that allows for the needed cooperative effort at healing. Resolution of parent-child versus adult-adult models in communication is further complicated by the inherent presence of patient regression in the health care setting; in order to survive in a hospital, a patient must regress, giving up the trappings of his adult and self-directed person and allowing others access to his body and its functionings. The double-bind of much of health care is that the patient is asked to be both the passive, compliant child/patient and to accept responsibility for his condition and to make decisions as an adult.

The effects of this conflict and double-bind upon doctor-patient communication can be profound, and it generally falls to the physician to resolve them through managing and structuring his interaction with the patient. To do this, the physician can employ a number of intervention techniques to facilitate adult-adult communication without compromising health care delivery. A hidden benefit for the doctor who is skilled in communications techniques is that he can use the communication process not only to educate the patient about his illness, thus reducing patient anxiety, but also educate the patient about communicating with doctors.

Limit-setting, mentioned earlier, is one of the techniques that can enhance doctor-patient communication. In limit-setting, one person in the interaction, most typically the physician, verbalizes controls upon the nature or extent of the communication interaction. An example of this would be when the doctor says, "I have just fifteen minutes to spend with you now, so let's deal with your most urgent questions; tomorrow I'll set aside more time so that we can get to the other questions you have." Limit-setting serves to clarify expectations and by doing so reduces anxiety or communication dissonance. Related to this technique is *partializing* in which one conveys the message "let's deal with one thing at a time." As medical care becomes more specialized, the ability to partialize becomes more important, especially in communicating with patients who suffer from complex medical problems where multiple specialists are involved. Few patient complaints are more common than the one in which the patient indicates that every doctor tells him something different. Partializing helps the patient both to understand the variations in information based on medical specialization and to direct his questions to the appropriate specialist.

Confronting is a third communication skill used by the doctor to enhance his communication with the patient, but it is a skill that requires judicious employment. Confronting means pointing out a maladaptive behavior that interferes either with the communication process or with the medical treatment, and its use is tied to the existence of an already existing, reasonably positive relationship with the patient. Confrontation cannot ordinarily be used in an initial doctor-patient contact. Whenever it is used, however, it requires a caring rather than an angry tone in order to be effective, because the inherent message in confrontation is "cut that out!" Thus the doctor might point out to the patient that each day she asks him the same questions or that she fails to follow medical recommendations or that she is in some way behaving in a manner that is unacceptable. If a physician uses confrontation in an angry, self-righteous manner, the ensuing doctor-patient communication will tend to become polar and mutually recriminative rather than cooperative, and it will be exceptionally difficult for both parties to retreat from this stance without losing an irremediable amount of "face."

Giving information is, without doubt, the most commonly employed intervention for guiding physician-patient communication. It requires a determination on the part of the doctor of what to say, how much to say, and when to say it. Misjudgment in these areas can lead the physician to say too much, too little, or to say whatever he says too soon or too late to enhance communication with the patient. Unlike prescribing the dosage of a drug, there is no clear formula for giving information, and consequently, it is a skill grounded in clinical judgment and physician self-awareness.

A major component of giving information is *educating* the patient about his condition with the goal of inspiring the patient to follow medical recommendations. The tacit contingency relationship of educating is that if a person understands what is wrong with him, then he will modify his behavior to resolve his illness in accordance with the physician's direction. The educative component of information giving also reduces ambiguity for the patient, resulting in lowered anxiety as well.

A second component of information giving is the skill of offering *direct advice*. In theory, it seems easy for one person, especially an ascribed expert, to tell another person what to do, but in practice, providing direct advice is a subtle technique as much based in the doctor's understanding and appreciation of latent factors as of manifest ones. Thus, when the physician sees an obese male patient who smokes two packs of cigarettes each day, never exercises, and works in a sedentary, executive position, the doctor may want to tell the patient to lose thirty pounds, quit smoking, and take up jogging, but in all likelihood, he will titrate his advice to the patient in accord with his recognition of the patient as a whole person as well as his knowledge of the potential or actual medical problems related to the patient's life-style. Generally speaking, direct advice is most likely to be followed if it is congruent with the patient's value system and if the rewards resulting from accepting the advice are clear. In cultures in which plumpness is defined as a feature of good health because it represents having food, or in cultures where plumpness is seen as a feature of female attractiveness or masculine strength, direct advice from a doctor to lose weight will not be well-received because cultural prescription supercedes medical prescription; if the physician does not know this, he may feel angry or frustrated by patient failure to follow his advice and his ability to communicate with the patient will be affected; but if he does know it, he may well have chosen not to mention weight loss as a goal, substituting more culturally acceptable advice instead.

Ultimately, the key to effective doctor-patient communication lies in semantics, in the ways the words of speech are chosen and used. Semantic choice involves both physician and patient; it exists as a fluid process, constantly being modified both consciously and unconsciously by both parties as they sense and respond to the cues that they receive of comprehension from the other half of the interaction. Technical versus common terminology, idiom, figures of speech, and humor are at issue here, for unless there is mutuality of semantic choice, communication is impaired, even if both doctor and patient are listening and speaking.

The patient often feels concern about revealing his ignorance to the physician, and this concern acts as a censor upon his use of language so that he withdraws from the communication process rather than embarrass himself by asking a question. Although most people have names for the external parts of their bodies and for some of their bodies' functions, many people live with a staggering lack of information about how their bodies are made. If asked to draw what their insides look like, they draw a sort of balloon in which viscera, blood, bones, and muscles float and slosh about virtually at random. In a supportive atmosphere, patients can sometimes verbalize these beliefs, such as the common fear that daily venipunctures for blood studies will deplete the body's blood supply or, as one woman said, that drinking orange juice would lead to burning on urination. Even relatively simple medical terminology—"fractured" as opposed to "broken"—is unknown to many patients.

The implication of this, then, is that the physician must somehow adjust his use of language to that comprehensible to the patient without, at the same time, making the patient feel patronized. This can be an extraordinarily difficult charge, and to assist in this aspect of communication, some doctors use simple drawings, three-dimensional models, pamphlets that the patient can keep, or include a less technical facilitator such as a social worker, nurse, or patient friend or relative who can serve as a pseudointerpreter for the patient and for the doctor as well.

In summary, physician-patient communication has been considered as a delicate and fluid process, fraught with imbalances and with semantic difficulties. Nonetheless, it is a process that can be enhanced through the physician's conscious use of himself, through efforts in medical education to train doctors in specific communications techniques, through the thoughtful employment of visual aids and reading materials, and by enlisting the help of professional or lay facilitators to serve as adjuncts and intermediaries in the communication process. The payoff for improved doctor-patient communication is the working partnership that is the foundation of good health care.

REFERENCES

Friedson, E. *Patients' Views of Medical Practice*. New York: Russell Sage Foundation, 1961.

Goffman, E. *The Presentation of Self in Everyday Life*. Garden City: Doubleday Anchor Books, 1959.

Goffman, E. *Frame Analysis: An Essay on the Organization of Experience*. Cambridge: Harvard University Press, 1974.

King, S. H. *Perceptions of Illness and Medical Practice*. New York: Russell Sage Foundation, 1962.

MacKinnon, R. A., and Michels, R. *The Psychiatric Interview in Clinical Practice*. Philadelphia: W. B. Saunders Co., 1971.

Middleman, R. R., and Goldberg, G. *Social Service Delivery: A Structural Approach to Social Work Practice*. New York: Columbia University Press, 1974.

University of Michigan School of Social Work. Instructional materials on the teaching of communication intervention skills (unpublished).

Section II

This section addresses specific aspects of communication that are unique to health care systems. The chapters emphasize that communication is not limited to the explicit content of verbal transactions in health care settings. The reader is reminded that such disparate items as furniture arrangement and medical records are important communicative tools. Once the perspective of potential communicators is broadened, approaches such as assertiveness training and audiovisual aids to improve communication skills can be utilized.

Chapter 5

LIABILITIES OF COMMUNICATION: INFORMED CONSENT—THE PATIENTS' AND PROFESSIONALS' RIGHTS AND DUTIES

Oliver Schroeder, Jr.

INTRODUCTION: FAITH, HEALTH AND JUSTICE

Human life on spaceship Earth is a continuous process which seeks to create a proper fusion of faith, health and justice. Our subject, "Liabilities of Communication: Informed Consent" represents a most acute contemporary experience in this process. A definition of each of these three basic ingredients of life is in order.

Faith is a belief in some supreme being. It may be God, Allah, or the "Creator" as described by lawyer Jefferson in the Declaration of Independence. Individual faith seeks to answer the truly profound questions of human life—What am I? Who am I? Why am I? Each individual must answer these questions to his own personal satisfaction whether he is a professional health care provider or a professional justice provider. In addition, the same needs in other persons must be recognized whether they are called patients or clients. The concept of faith is not to be taken lightly. In 1978, as humanity approaches the 1980s, faith with its three profound questions may well be the most important concept confronting mankind.

Health, on the other hand, has best been defined by the World Health Organization. "Health is the state of physical, mental and social well-being." Medical physicians and allied health professionals, e.g. dentists, nurses, psychologists, social workers, etc., are workers in the constant effort to achieve, restore, and maintain that state of well-being for the individual person as well as for the whole human family.

Finally, justice is that relationship between and among human beings seeking to assure peace, order, security, and happiness for each individual. Justice is based on a proper mixture of fairness, reasonableness, equity, justness, impartiality and uniformity. Law with its professionals, e.g. lawyers, judges, legislators, public executives and administrators, is a tool to achieve, restore, and maintain the properly balanced relationship that is called justice.

In America, law is not the only tool to obtain justice for individuals and the whole community. Moral principles drawn from religious precepts founded on individual faith are constantly infused into the administration of justice. Some individuals have that abundant faith and physical strength to stand up for a better justice. Dr. Martin Luther King, Jr. deliberately violated the law in Birmingham, Alabama. He intentionally sought arrest, willingly went to jail, and from his jail cell sent forth his remarkable epistle to America, "A Letter from the Birmingham Jail." This act of faith helped dramatically to change the legal relationships between black and white Americans. By using a foundation of faith to undergird moral action, he thereby changed the law to achieve a higher justice for every human being.

THE SPINAL CORD INJURY PATIENT

How do these concepts of faith, health, and justice fit into the care and treatment of the spinal cord injured? In today's world, especially in America, the patient seeking the maximum state of well-being in health has been discovering and responding to these basic questions of faith—What am I? Who am I? Why am I? The patient now believes that he is a free and equal human being with every other person; that he is a partner with the professional health care practitioner to achieve his healthy state of personal well-being. The patient does not see himself as a serf to be handled by a sovereign—the professional health care provider. In the medical question of what is to be done to or for the patient, the patient is now the managing partner. He has that ultimate human right—the right of self-determination—when it is his health care, his diagnosis or his treatment which is being considered or handled. Today this relationship is emerging as the acceptable level for personal justice. The law is responding with new actions to achieve this justice: the law of informed consent or the right of self-determination.

HISTORY OF INFORMED CONSENT

Where did the legal concepts of informed consent begin? In 1905, the Minnesota Supreme Court promulgated in *Mohr v. Williams,*

> Under a free government, at least, the free citizen's first and greatest right, which underlies all others,—the right to the inviolability of his person, in other words, the right to himself—is the subject of universal acquiescence, and this right necessarily forbids a physician and surgeon, however skillful or eminent . . . to violate, without permission, the bodily integrity of his patient . . . [1]
> The patient must be the final arbiter as to whether he will take his chance with the operation, or take his chances of living without it. Such is the natural right of the individual, which the law recognizes as a legal right.[2]
> If [the defendent's act] was unauthorized, then it was, within what we have said, unlawful. It was a violent assault, not a mere pleasantry, and even though no negligence is shown, it was wrongful, and unlawful. The case is unlike a criminal prosecution for assault and battery, for there an unlawful intent must be shown. But that rule does not apply to a civil action, to maintain which it is sufficient to show that the assault complained of was wrongful and unlawful or the result of negligence.[3]

While the legal liability of the health care provider is firmly fixed where informed consent has not been obtained, the Minnesota Supreme Court did recognize the right of the health care practitioner to show any benefit provided the patient and the good faith of the practitioner. Legally these two mitigating circumstances permit the jury to lower the amount of damages awarded to the patient for injuries received as the result of no informed consent being given.

A second celebrated case in the growth of informed consent law was *Schloendorff v. New York Hospital* decided in 1914. Chief Justice Benjamin N. Cardozo of the New York Court of Appeals wrote:

> Every human being of adult years and sound mind has a right to determine what shall be done with his own body; and a surgeon who performs an operation without his patient's consent, commits an assault, for which he is liable in damages. This is true except in cases of emergency where the patient is unconscious and where it is necessary to operate before consent can be obtained.[4]

The basic concepts of the patient's right to self-determination have developed consistently along the lines set forth in *Mohr* and *Schloendorff*. In 1960 the Kansas Supreme Court in writing in *Natanson v. Kline* further stated:

> [E]ach man is considered to be the master of his own body, and he may, if he be of sound mind, expressly prohibit the performance of life-saving surgery, or other medical treatment. A doctor might well believe that an operation or form of treatment is desirable or necessary but the law does not permit him to substitute his own judgment for that of the patient by any form or artifice or deception.[5]

These three landmark cases and numerous other decisions in almost every jurisdiction have provided by 1978 a large body of informed consent law.

WHAT IS INFORMED CONSENT?

Today, without proper two-way communications to provide opportunity for intelligent, informed, voluntary self-determination, the provider of diagnosis, treatment and care can be subjected by law to both civil and criminal liabilities. The concept of justice in the area of the patient's informed consent has been elevated in the past two decades. The legal action now available to patients to achieve this new justice relationship is termed a battery, civil, or criminal. A battery is simply an *unlawful* touching of another person. If it is done intentionally and maliciously, it is a crime. Even if it is done without malice and with the best of intentions (to provide better health for the victim) it is still a civil wrong. Why? Because the patient has the right of self-determination based upon information which permits him to make an intelligent and reasonable consent to the health professional's touching him for diagnosis, care or treatment.

To avoid liability for a battery, civil or criminal, the health professional should follow this procedure:

> The patient must be told in language he understands: (1) the diagnosis, (2) the nature of the prescribed procedure to be performed, (3) the risks, complications, and benefits involved, (4) the prognosis if the treatment is not carried out, (5) alternative methods of treatment (if any) (6) that the patient is free to withdraw his consent at any time.

If this exemplary procedure is followed, the patient is held by law to have given his valid consent—both informed and voluntary. As long as these six elements are present, the consent may be either oral or written. If oral, a written notation of such should be placed in the patient's medical record and initialed by the health care provider who obtained the oral consent.

In some states, the elements of consent are established by statute, but generally they are established by case law which is judicial decision law. If research or experimental procedures are used, or new techniques utilized, some jurisdictions require that the consent be in writing and signed by the patient. Written consents are always preferable, since the writing provides excellent proof of the patient's consent.

Where federal financial assistance is used for reseach on human subjects, the U.S. Department of Health, Education and Welfare guidelines require that an informed consent be obtained. The guidelines also require that it be in writing and signed by the patient. When research is carried out in an institutional setting, such as in a university, hospital, health center, or dental clinic, the institutional rules as well as state laws, or governmental administrative regulations concerning informed consent, must be understood and followed in order to protect the institution, the patient, and the health care providers.

A rapid development of the institutional informed consent rules has been occurring. In such institutional settings the persons who practice health care should not only become familiar with the present rules, but more importantly watch for changes.

The trend in the whole informed consent law area—federal laws and regulations, state statutes, case law, institutional rules—has been to restrict severely the latitude of the health practitioner's care in relation to the patient's legal rights. More specificity in informing patients of the risks involved in a particular diagnosis, treatment, or care is being required. Written and signed consents are being mandated. Voluntary decisions by an understanding patient are expected.

WHAT LEGAL RIGHTS AND DUTIES EXIST IN THE INFORMED CONSENT AREA?

As judicial decisions on informed consent have grown in number over the decades, the situations involving this legal issue have generally appeared under these conditions: a total lack of consent by the patient, failure to obtain the proper consent in the care of minors, consent which is too vague, extension of care beyond that area to which consent has been given, performance of care different from that for which the consent was obtained, obtaining consent based upon inadequate information provided the patient, and consent given involuntarily.

At the same time the courts have eased certain restrictions in this legal area. The courts have implied an informed consent in certain situations: the patient goes to a health clinic on a day set aside for vaccination; he stands in line and watches others being vaccinated; when his turn comes he proceeds to do likewise; no words of explanation were given to the person; no words of consent were issued by patient; but, the law will imply that the patient gave an informed consent based on the patient's actions under such a situation.

Consent has also been implied by law without the patient's issuing any words of consent. A patient, who is under a general anesthetic for surgery and an unanticipated need arises to extend that surgery beyond the original area of consent, is presumed by law to give consent because a reasonably prudent person in such a situation would do so. The North Carolina Supreme Court in 1956 in *Kennedy v. Parrott,*[6] set the following conditions for implying such consent as a matter of law: (1) the condition encountered cannot reasonably have been diagnosed prior to surgery; (2) the surgery in question has not been expressly proscribed by the patient; (3) the more extensive surgery is in the area of the original incision; (4) sound medical practice dictates such an extension; and (5) neither the patient nor a surrogate is immediately available to give the necessary consent.

A major question for all health care professionals is who can give an informed consent. Consent can be legally given by a patient who is:
1. Eighteen years of age or older
2. An emancipated minor (sixteen years or older living away from home)
3. A mature minor (fifteen years or older who understands his health problems)

Note that most minors and mental incompetents cannot give consent. A parent, guardian, or court must provide legal consent for these patients.

Equally important is who should obtain the consent. The person who is to provide the diagnosis, care, or treatment must obtain the consent. No agent can be delegated this duty. He who touches the patient's body must get the patient's consent.

RESEARCH AND INNOVATIVE TECHNIQUES

If the patient is one upon whom research or experiments are being conducted, federal regulations and institutional rules, in addition to the usual informed and voluntary consent law, will apply:
1. A fair explanation of the procedures to be followed and their purposes including an identification of any procedures that are experimental.
2. A description of the attendant discomforts and risks.
3. A description of the benefits to be expected. With nonbeneficial research there should be a clear statement indicating that the research is not of benefit to the subject. In addition, the benefit to society and the group that may benefit from the investigation should be indicated to the subject.
4. A disclosure of appropriate alternative procedures that might be advantageous for the subject.
5. An offer to answer any inquiries concerning the procedures.

6. An instruction that the subject is free to withdraw his consent and to discontinue participation in the project or activity at any time without prejudice to the subject.

When medical research or experimentation is to be done on minors, pregnant women, prisoners, or mentally retarded or mentally disabled persons, very stringent legal restrictions are often applied. Great care with legal counseling in such situations is most wise.

The courts take a different approach when considering new, innovative techniques that have clearly developed beyond the experimental stage. Since the modern interpretation of informed consent includes the need to identify alternative methods of treatment, courts will accept the fact that differences in opinion as to the values of alternative treatment procedures occur among health practitioners. In establishing standards of care relative to deciding cases of alleged malpractice in new and innovative technique cases, the courts have accepted those new treatment techniques which have been approved by a respectable minority of the medical community. Thus, the courts have not discouraged innovation in health practice. Where these latter principles apply, special provisions need not be included in the consent agreement.

SPECIAL CONCERNS IN SPINAL CORD INJURIES

The law recognizes spinal cord injuries as very serious matters in the medicolegal area. No better evidence of this concern is the dollar value placed on such injuries. For the six-month period, July–December, 1977, a private reporting system, by no means including all verdicts, awards, or settlements in the United States, indicated that the dollar values assigned in spinal cord injury cases where civil liability existed ranged up to $9,341,683 for a single case. Of the twenty-three cases reported, ten cases had dollar values exceeding $1,000,000.

A second special concern in this type of injury involves the division for separating the customary care for spinal cord injury patients from new, innovative care and in like manner the separation of new, innovative care from research or experimental care. The nature of spinal cord injuries invites new innovations as well as pure research or experiment. The practitioners must be sensitive to these categories and determine in which legal area they are functioning.

Thirdly, spinal cord injury cases demand the most intense provider-patient communication and highest mutual trust. Psychologically, to both parties, the patient's self-determination right can be a most valuable health asset, not just a legal requirement.

Finally, because of the very extreme personal injury represented by spinal cord injuries, the law will place the utmost legal demands on the health care provider; hence, the informed consent procedures provided in such cases will be more carefully scrutinized by judges and lawyers.

CONCLUSIONS

The health professional must satisfy legal requirements in obtaining informed consent from patients in all professional endeavors. Recognition of the patient's right to self-determination is the first step. Establishment of routine consent procedures, either oral or written, is next. Finally, the actual voluntary consent of the patient to a certain course of diagnosis, care, or treatment must be obtained. This consent must be based upon the patient's informed understanding of the diagnosis, care or treatment, the nature of the prescribed procedure, the risks and complications involved in the treatment as well as the benefits that may result, the prognosis of care or treatment. A most valuable by-product of this legal, professional procedure is often the enhancement of the professional provider-patient relationship. The clarification of the expectations of both parties concerning the delivery of professional services is a factor that will also reduce exposure to malpractice charges. The law of informed consent not only ensures the patient's right to determine what course of diagnosis, care, or treatment is to be undertaken, it also elevates the professionalism of every health care practitioner.

REFERENCES

1. 95 *Minnesota Reports* 261, 268; 104 *Northwestern Reporter* 12, 14.
2. 95 *Minnesota Reports* 261, 268 and 15.
3. 95 *Minnesota Reports* 261, 271 and 16.
4. 211 *New York Reports* 125, 129-130; 105 *Northeastern Reporter* 92, 93.
5. 186 *Kansas Reports* 393, 406-407; 350 *Pacific Reporter* 2nd 1093, 1104.
6. 243 *North Carolina Reports* 355; 90 *Southeastern Reporter* 2nd 754.

Chapter 6

ASSERTIVE BEHAVIOR IN HEALTH CARE SETTINGS

Barbara E. Yocum

The self-help movement has taken many forms over the past decade. It has moved from very loose sensitivity group activity to very structured types of behavior modification. Each form has had its own disciples and practitioners, and each has benefitted some people in its own way.

No matter what form of self-help is undertaken, problems can develop when the person, with his/her new self-understanding or skills, moves back into old settings and into normal routines of work, home, and social life. Seldom does there exist support or even understanding for the changes in behaviors that may have occurred. In a nonsupportive setting, new behaviors may be lost before they are developed enough to have a positive effect on the individual's role in that setting.

It is with concern for organizational influence on behavior change that this chapter is written. Merely addressing assertiveness as a means of improving interpersonal effectiveness and self-concept is not enough. It is also necessary to address the characteristics and influences of the health care setting in order to give meaning to the practice of assertive behavior for health care professionals.

Definitions

When we interact with another person, we have a choice of responses and reactions. We can be harsh and demanding, quiet, low-key, passive, manipulative, teasing, or confrontive. We can react spontaneously and naturally, or with conditioned responses of guilt, suspicion, hostility, fear, or nervous laughter. In assertiveness training this multitude of responses is categorized into three types of behavior: *assertive, aggressive,* and *nonassertive* or *passive* behaviors. (The term "unassertive" will be used when referring to both aggressive and nonassertive behaviors.)

Assertive behavior is described as interpersonal behavior that is an honest, direct, and appropriate expression of one's feelings, beliefs, or needs. Assertiveness shows a balance of respect for oneself and one's personal rights with respect for others and their rights. It involves communicating one's own position while remaining aware of the other person's needs or wishes. Honest communication, self-disclosure, limit-setting, and negotiating for compromise are goals of assertive behavior.

Some specific examples of assertive behavior include giving compliments or opinions, expressing disagreement, and asking for information or clarification. Assertive statements are accompanied by appropriate physical behavior, such as direct eye contact, steady voice, and centered, natural body posture.

The meaning of assertive behavior becomes clearer when contrasted with aggressive and nonassertive styles. While aggressive behavior may also be considered direct and honest, it typically lacks consideration or respect for other persons and their rights. Harsh criticism, displaced anger, put-downs, and superiority are characteristic aggressive expressions. Aggression involves trying to get one's way or winning through domination, humiliation, or manipulation. Such behavior often induces guilt or fear in the other person. It is accompanied by physical actions such as demanding or accusatory tones of voice, staring or glaring, waving arms, or pounding fists. Aggressive behavior is typically inappropriate, often an overreaction to a situation.

Persons displaying nonassertive or passive behavior often become the victims of aggressive persons by failing to stand up for their rights and failing to make their own needs known. They may express themselves in such an indirect or apologetic manner that they are not heard. Thus, they often allow others to decide or make choices for them.

Anxiety over possible consequences or fear of what others might think are feelings that underlie nonassertive behavior. There is a need to appease others and avoid conflict and disapproval. Nonassertive persons place their own self-respect far below respect for others. Physical characteristics include downcast or averted eyes, soft or hesitant tone of voice, or generally anxious demeanor.

In reviewing the many theoretical and practical approaches to assertive training, Alberti (1977) suggests a perspective that states:
 (1) Assertiveness is a characteristic of *behavior*, not of *persons*.
 (2) Assertiveness is a *person-and-situation* specific, not a universal characteristic.
 (3) Assertiveness must be viewed in the *cultural context* of the individual, as well as in terms of other situational variables.
 (4) Assertiveness is predicated on the ability of the individual to *freely choose* his/her action.
 (5) Assertiveness is a characteristic of *socially effective, nonhurtful* behavior.

This perspective indicates that most of us are faced with various *situations* in which we are dissatisfied with our behaviors. For example, one may be comfortably assertive with one friend, but passive with another. Or, passive behavior may be shown in the office, while kicking the dog releases aggression at home. Certain personality types may evoke particular responses that are not the norm. Particular atmospheres, such as an important social function, may cause anxiety in a normally calm person. There are some people who are generally aggressive or passive, of course. But most of the normal population face *situational* unassertiveness. Let us review the primary blocks that prevent us from acting assertively in health care situations.

Blocks to Assertive Behavior

The primary block to behaving assertively is the collection of "shoulds," "oughts," "don'ts," and "what will happen if's" that most people carry with them. Messages from family, school, social environment, and work settings shape perception of how one ought to be or act. Especially influential messages are ones like: "Take care of others first," "Don't show your feelings," "Be a lady (man)," "Never trust anyone you don't know," and "Don't get involved."

Part of becoming an adult is giving oneself permission to continue developing—to sort out and discard inappropriate "shoulds." Unfortunately, some messages are so strongly ingrained that they become an unconscious part of life. As a result, many adults, self-sufficient in other areas, continue to function interpersonally from childhood or adolescent messages that are never recognized or confronted.

Some of these messages are reinforced in the workplace. In the health care setting, there is a traditional hierarchy of authority, from physician to nurse to support staff to patient. This hierarchy can reinforce messages like "Know your place," "Don't question authority," and "Do what you're told."

Each level of the hierarchy has its own set of messages that can interfere in interpersonal effectiveness.

PHYSICIANS. Physician's messages are developed early and reinforced throughout their education and training. Some of the more common forms are "Be perfect," "Don't show any emotion," and "Stay in control."

NURSES. Many of those who enter the nursing profession are guided by messages such as "Give, give, give," "Take care of others," "Put others first," and "Be humble, never brag or complain."

NURSING ASSISTANTS. Many of the nursing messages can also work for nursing assistants. Others, such as "I'm only an assistant," "Know your place," and "Respect those above you," also come into play.

PATIENTS. Patients bring messages from personal life that influence their hospital behavior. However, depending on their level of illness, typical messages are "I'm helpless," "No one cares that I'm sick (dying, in pain, etc.,") and "I'm scared."

Add to these three groups the interactions of hospital and staff administrators, technicians, therapists, family and friends, ward clerks, housekeeping staff, and all the other groups necessary for a hospital to function. A picture of the complexities of human interaction develops very clearly.

On top of these messages are others about working, whatever the occupation. Messages like "Work hard and you'll get your reward," "Never refuse a request for help, whatever it costs you" are common. Supervisors often have messages about staying in control

("I'm the only one who knows what's going on here") or giving compliments ("Don't praise them—it'll just go to their heads").

In unsatisfactory situations, a person may take a passive approach of "There's nothing I can do about it anyway." Others take an aggressive approach by causing trouble at every turn but never working to rectify or improve the situation.

The impact such messages have on our behavior is so significant that they can keep us acting out old behaviors that we may not even like. A primary part of learning assertive skills is confronting our own strong messages, and sorting out the positive from the negative. Then we can determine for ourselves which messages are appropriate for now, to help us modify behaviors and situations with which we are dissatisfied.

Interpersonal Rights

We can begin to confront the irrationality of messages by building a set of counteracting positive beliefs. Fundamental to the practice of assertive behavior is the belief that we have the *right* to be assertive. Jakubowski (1976) proposes two basic beliefs. First, assertion—rather than manipulation, submission, or hostility—enriches life, and ultimately leads to more satisfying personal relationships. Secondly, everyone is entitled to act assertively, and to express honest thoughts, feelings, and beliefs.

Many more specific human rights can be developed from these two basic beliefs. Examples include the right to have and express our needs, to ask for help, to have and express feelings, to make mistakes, to decide for ourselves. Underlying these rights is the accompanying *responsibility* of not violating the rights of others while expressing our own rights.

By identifying and accepting these rights for ourselves, we can give ourselves permission to sort out the old, irrational messages and replace them with new thoughts about assertive behavior.

Example:

Old Message	Assertive Message
The doctor will think I'm stupid if I ask what this order means.	I'd rather ask and give the medication than guess and be wrong.

I wouldn't be much of a friend if I didn't work Jane's shift for her Saturday night. I'm not really doing anything important anyway. I'll guess I'll do it.	If it were an emergency I would help Jane out. But my time is really important this weekend. Jane knows me well enough to understand.

Accepting these new thoughts lays the groundwork for moving into assertive behaviors. We feel more comfortable asking for clarification or refusing a request when we believe that we have the right to do so.

Developing Assertive Behaviors

The process of developing assertive behaviors begins with identifying specific situations that cause discomfort or difficulty. It is necessary to start with small steps when learning any new skill. Likewise it is important to start with small situations that are less threatening or difficult to modify.

Determining the messages and emotions that the situation evokes is next. Having a firm understanding of messages, fears, and feelings can begin to clarify the behaviors that need changing.

Creating positive messages to replace the old is the third step. Restructuring our thoughts on the basis of our rights leads us to a healthier belief system.

With new messages firmly in mind, we can begin to develop assertive statements and physical behaviors in front of a mirror, with a tape recorder, in a fantasy, or with a supportive friend. Then apply your practical skills to the real situation.

Example: Confrontation with Co-workers—Setting Limits

Situation: Co-worker is slow in completing her work. She asks you to help her. At first you didn't mind, but it's become an everyday happening. You're getting tired of doing her work for her.

Old Messages	*Assertive Messages*
Don't rock the boat or cause trouble.	It's true that the patients' care is important. But I can't give good care if I have too much to do

The patients' care is more important than our personal squabbles.	because of her slowness.
	I have the right to refuse her requests for help, so that I can do my job better.
She might make trouble for me if I get angry with her.	
The supervisor is sure to notice pretty soon, and she'll take care of it.	The issue is between the two of us. If we handle it, then the supervisor won't get involved. The trouble will stop with us, rather than going higher up.

Assertive Statement: Mary, our work situation has begun to bother me. I did agree to help you with baths on Monday, but now you're asking me to do more every day. I can't give my patients good care if I have to do some of your work too. I will share some of my methods of getting things done quickly with you. Maybe that will help you. If not, you might want to talk to the supervisor about changing your patient load.

Situational Implications

There are implications for assertive behavior at all levels within the health care setting. Two specific developments have particular impact. One is the growing emphasis on consumerism and patient rights. It is increasingly common for patients to move from the role of helpless child to that of involved adult. Expectations from the health care system have changed. Patients ask for and expect clear information and explanations. "Because the doctor says so" is no longer an acceptable reason for a treatment. Assertive skills can give both patients and staff confidence in handling issues related to patient rights.

Secondly, moving from a structured hierarchy to a team approach for medical treatment has forced changes in staff relationships. A structure of Doctor-Nurse-Therapist-Aide-Patient provides security, a set of rules that dictate behavior. Decisions and choices are few for staff and for patients.

However, when information from a dietician, an aide, or a therapist is equally as important as that from a doctor, the dynamics change. Old messages of "My opinion doesn't count" or "I don't know as much as they do," or "I'm the expert here" are no longer valid, and interfere in the success of the team. Using assertive behaviors can increase individual self-confidence as well as enhance the team's effectiveness in working together.

For patients, learning assertive behaviors can assist in reducing fears about their illness, in learning to live with new limits, and in restructuring relationships to meet new needs.

For hospital staff members at all levels, assertiveness can help clarify issues, set limits, confront problems and generally operate more successfully within a changing, stressful environment.

For persons in management, assertive skills can assist in handling managerial tasks such as staffing and evaluation, as well as in related personal career issues.

Summary

Assertiveness is not a universal panacea for instant change. To bring significant, lasting change to an organization, a commitment to training for all levels of staff would be the ideal. A broad training program would provide an atmosphere of support and encouragement for the continued development of interpersonal skills and teamwork.

However, learning assertive behaviors can increase personal effectiveness in single individuals, who then feel more self-confident about working to make their immediate surroundings more productive.

The effects of assertiveness training have been compared to the ripples from a pebble thrown in a pond. A change in one person's behavior can impact on many others in unknown ways. In a health care environment, where the primary goal is contributing to human wellness, it is important that health care workers take care of themselves and their associates so they can give quality care to others. Developing assertive behaviors can make a significant contribution to a healthy health environment.

REFERENCES

Alberti, R. I. (Ed.). *Assertiveness: Innovations, Applications, Issues.* San Luis Obispo: Impact Pubs. Inc., 1977.

Alberti, R. E., and Emmons, M. L. *Your Perfect Right: A Guide to Assertive Behavior.* San Luis Obispo: Impact Pubs. Inc., 1970.

Alberti, R. E., and Emmons, M. L. *Stand Up, Speak Out, Talk Back!* New York: Pocket Books, 1975.

Bloom, L., Coburn, K., and Pearlman, J. *The New Assertive Woman.* New York: Delacorte Press, 1975.

Bower, S., and Bower, G. *Asserting Yourself: A Practical Guide for Positive Change.* Menlo Park: Addison-Wesley Publishers, 1976.

Fensterheim, H., and Boyer, J. *Don't Say Yes When You Want to Say No.* New York: David McKay Publishers, 1975.

Jongeward, D., and Scott, D. *Women as Winners.* Menlo Park, California: Addison-Wesley Publishing Co., Inc., 1976.

Lange, A., and Jakubowski, P. *Responsible Assertive Behavior: Cognitive and Behavioral Procedures for Trainers.* Champaign, Illinois: Research Press, 1976.

Lazarus, A., and Fay, A. *I Can If I Want To.* New York: Morrow Publishing Co. 1975.

Phelps, S., and Austin, N. *The Assertive Woman.* San Luis Obispo: Impact Pubs. Inc., 1975.

Chapter 7

NONVERBAL COMMUNICATION

Elizabeth Wales

The important thing to remember about nonverbal behaviors is that they are *learned* and that their function is to *communicate*. In order to be communicative both the actor emitting the behavior and the person perceiving the behavior must share the same understanding as to the "meaning" of that behavior. People seem fascinated by nonverbal behavior because it seems to tell them things they didn't know about themselves and others. Yet, how can this be, if we all learned it and share a common understanding as to its meaning?

This seeming paradox occurs because these behaviors are ones we have learned without their having been taught. They are truly out-of-awareness behaviors. They shape and influence our interactions with others, but usually we attribute the behavior of ourselves and others to more conscious dynamics of motivations. These nonverbal behaviors of learned and shared meaning are based on the norms of the various social, cultural, or ethnic groups in which we have been raised and to which we belong. Generally, when you review the literature on nonverbal behaviors, the findings are based on white, middle-class American groups. To the extent that you belong to that group the following nonverbal behaviors may be true of you. To the extent that you deviate from that group they will not be true of you.

It is useful to recognize nonverbal communication and its meaning as influenced by group norms, because typically we interpret (attribute) nonverbal behaviors that are different than our own as "pathology." For example, members of Jewish culture of Middle European background typically stand closer to each other and use more gestures and emotionally expressive body language than do Gentile middle-class white Americans. Suppose a Jewish patient of the type described engages in a conversation with his WASP physician. The physician is likely to leave that encounter thinking, "What a pushy, aggressive fellow. Highly excitable too, probably hysterical!" The patient on the other hand is likely to leave the encounter thinking, "What a cold, indifferent fellow. He doesn't care about me at all."

Both participants are right and both participants are wrong. They are "right" because if someone of their own group had responded to them with those same nonverbal behaviors, their attribution of the meaning of those behaviors would have been correct. They are "wrong" because they fail to recognize that they belong to different groups in which nonverbal behaviors have different meanings.

Besides the importance of recognizing group membership in understanding nonverbal communication, it is equally important to recognize the *context* in which the behavior takes place. The context must always be considered because frequently we only know the meaning of a bit of nonverbal behavior because it is a deviation from a particular base rate of norms of one's behavior. Many couples develop their own language in this way. Suppose you have a couple in which the husband always slams the door when he leaves in the morning. The morning he closes the door quietly his wife will think "oh, oh, something's wrong with him." Perhaps in your own experience you have met someone who has a serious, nonsmiling demeanor and you initially thought they were unfriendly or unhappy. Usually, you have repeated experiences of that person, you "learn" that is their normal demeanor, i.e. it doesn't mean what it usually means in other people, and you can easily tell when they are actually unhappy or unfriendly by the changes from their usual norm. There are no universally true meanings for any piece of behavior.

People who are known for being "perceptive" are, I believe, people who are sensitive to nonverbal communications and perhaps most importantly, interpret it correctly. All of us can increase the accuracy of our reading of nonverbal communications and hence our perceptiveness if we become more aware of some of the determinants of their meaning by such factors as group membership and context.

Space

Hall (1969) identified four spatial distances that influence or are used for different social interactions.

INTIMATE SPACE. This is when two people stand either face touching face or up to six to eighteen inches apart. Physical touching is quite easy at this distance, eyes are slightly out of focus because of the nearness, at best you can only look at one eye or the other. At this distance you are probably either loving or fighting. Occasionally people are forced into this intimate distance when they are neither loving or fighting, i.e. when it is inappropriate, and we devise ways to negate the implied intimacy.

In crowded elevators we all stand facing the same way, elevate our eyes to watch the indicator to avoid catching anyone's gaze, and pull ourselves in to avoid touching. If you should doubt the power of nonverbal communication, try entering a crowded elevator and face the "wrong" way and look the person you are facing in the eye. If you survive to reach your destination, you will quickly become convinced that people are aware of correct and incorrect nonverbal behavior, interpret incorrect behavior as pathology and take immediate steps to correct the situation.

Interestingly, a good deal of medical practice is conducted at intimate distance and again we find ways of minimizing the intimacy and making the contact "appropriate." Talking briskly and matter-of-factly is one way, avoiding eye contact is another, and generally holding or carrying one's own body in a "professional" manner usually completes the process.

Another way we protect ourselves is with what Scheflen (1965) has called "barrier" behavior. "Barrier" behavior is when we literally place a physical barrier between ourselves and someone who is "inappropriately" close to us. It might be a hand raised to the head that creates an arm acting as a wall between ourselves and someone seated too close to us. Or it might consist of a leg crossed with a hand resting on the upraised knee that again creates a physical barrier between ourselves and the next person. Both actions clearly indicate the demarcation between our space and self from the other.

PERSONAL DISTANCE. According to Hall, personal distance can range from eighteen inches up to four feet. At this distance, which is about arm's length, touching is natural and easy should one want to touch. Conversation takes place in a fairly low tone which can be personal without being intimate. Invading this space by stepping too close makes people uncomfortable, often with their being unaware of why they are uncomfortable. When imposed upon in this way people will try to correct the situation by backing away. The next time you are having a conversation with a colleague try taking a step "too close." You might find you have backed your colleague down the length of the hall if you step too close; pause for them to adjust the distance to the "proper" space, then step too close again.

A nurse once told me about her supervisor who made her uncomfortable by standing too close. She "naturally" would adjust the distance to one that was more comfortable for her. Finally her supervisor would reach out and grab her arm to keep her from backing away from what, for the supervisor, was a comfortable speaking distance. These two women obviously had different norms of appropriate conversational space.

Besides the subculture influence of ethnic group membership, other factors affect spacing. Henley (1977) has described how we tend to give greater space to higher status. Certainly higher status goes with bigger offices, bigger homes, bigger desks, and greater space in general. For example, if four people are standing waiting for an elevator and one of them is the boss and the other three are his subordinates you will likely see the three subordinates standing fairly close together but clearly separated from the boss, almost as if he had a circle of authority about him.

High status males are often easily identified in groups. Watch at your next staff meeting and you are likely to see the high status male take the best seat in the room, however the best seat is defined in that setting; either by location, comfort, size, or some combination. As Goffman (1971) has noted, once seated, the high status male will have a relaxed, expansive body position while males of lesser status will sit with more body tension and attentiveness. Occasionally the high status male will throw back his shoulders with coat open, insert his thumbs in the top of his trousers with arms akimbo with an expansive display of chest. A display a lower status male would be very uncomfortable doing in the presence of a higher status male.

Another factor is sex role, whether one is male or female. Males in general have and take more space than females. Sex role may be confounded by status, however, as males generally have more status in our society than do females. Henley (1977) in a chapter entitled "The Incredible Shrinking Woman" cites many studies illustrating this difference between male and female use of space. Besides having more space, males invade females' space more often than the reverse.

Women are trained as part of being "nice" or "ladylike" to hold their arms and legs close in to their bodies, to condense. The next time you spend some time in a waiting room notice the difference in the positions of the males and females. You'll probably see the men sprawl, with spread legs, arms stretched across chairs or legs stretched out into the room. The women will more likely be sitting with their knees close together or legs crossed tightly together with their arms folded across their chest or wrapped around their pocketbook. The condensed body space is so much a part of females being nice or ladylike that a woman who is physically loose with her body arouses suspicions that she is indeed a "loose" woman.

Another factor that affects personal space is noticeable physical disability. A series of studies by Kleck (1969) showed that people tend to stand at greater distance from the obviously handicapped, but that the distance between them decreased the longer the two interact.

SOCIAL DISTANCE. Social distance can range from four to twelve feet. A great deal of our working and social relationships are conducted in this range. No touch is expected at this distance and eye contact is important. In fact, at the outer range, if there is no eye contact there is uncertainty whether or not you are still relating to that person. At that distance you could continue to work in the presence of another person and not be rude if you didn't acknowledge their presence with conversation.

There is some suggestion that blacks are different from whites in that they utilize verbal cues as well as visual contact to maintain an interaction. For example, at a social gathering white men will tend to form a circle or arc while conversing to facilitate eye contact, but black men may stand in a straight line while conversing and maintain contact by verbal responses such as "yeah," "that's right," "uh hum." Black preachers will tell you that if they did not get verbal responses from their parishioners during their sermon they would think they were in serious trouble with their congregations.

PUBLIC DISTANCE. Public distance ranges from twelve to twenty-five feet or more, if for example, one is a speaker on a stage. Public distance is so far apart that one must literally expand to reach across the space. Voices become louder, more formal; body movements become larger to communicate meaning. One in some sense becomes an actor, which is why some people never become comfortable with public distance. They often feel they "can't be themselves," that is, the way they are at closer distances.

Hall (1969), besides describing these four distances goes on to point out that the distance we position ourselves in relation to another is very much dependent on the nature of the action to be conducted, the relationship we have to the other, and how we feel about each other. Furthermore, this use of space is true for animals as well as for man.

Institutional Space

Besides the distance between people, which to some degree we control, the physical space, the environment around us, also influences our behavior and feelings. It is a truism to say that we behave in different ways according to the settings. Obviously, our party behavior is different than our work setting behavior.

Hospital rooms have in the past been sterile, foreign places which alter people's behavior by making them feel intimidated, helpless, and anxious. More recently attempts have been made to make hospital space more homelike, friendly in its setting, to encourage more normal patient behavior.

The use of space in the physical environment can pull people apart or bring them together. Either might be desirable in certain circumstances, but it would be well to be aware of when to do which.

Waiting rooms, for example, traditionally have been designed in a manner that tends to keep people apart. Seating arrangements are usually in a straight row; more recently, architects and interior decorators of institutional space have recognized that waiting rooms often involve periods of stress for the people in them and have begun to plan seating arrangements that pull people together, such as grouping of seats spaced throughout the waiting room. Occasionally you will still see in hospital day rooms or visiting areas chairs stiffly lined up around the walls. While this gives a neat appearance and is easy to maintain, after visiting hours or use by patients it is quite likely you'll find the chairs moved into semicircles—that is, if the chairs are movable at all. This is often a source of irritation to the nursing staff who keep "cleaning up" the area.

The positioning of the desk between doctor and patient can make a significant difference in the patient's behavior. White (1953) found that when a desk was placed between the doctor and patient which created a barrier only 10 percent of the patients were at ease. When the seating was rearranged so that the desk was not between the doctor and patient, up to 55 percent were perceived as at ease.

Osmond (1959), a director of a health and research center in Canada, found that the typical hospital arrangements of beds and furniture tended to separate the patients and resulted in less conversation between patients and increased depression. When the furniture was rearranged to encourage patient interaction, the amount of conversation increased and depression decreased.

Hospital rooms which are typically small can, by the arrangement of the furniture in them, give patients the feeling of being crowded and cramped or the experience of having enough room. Hall has pointed out that arrangement B is such that one can hardly move about without bumping in to something.

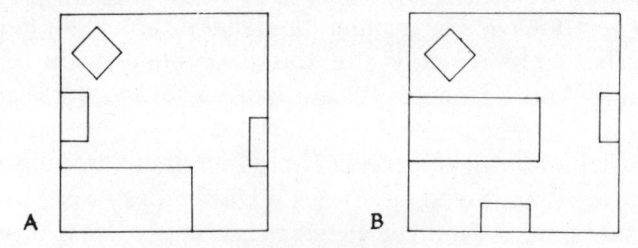

Figure 7-1. Arrangement of hospital furniture can alter the perception of physical space. In B, patients feel cramped; A gives the visual feeling of space.

People will often feel irritable and cramped in such an arrangement even though the physical dimensions are exactly the same as in arrangement A. The difference is that arrangement A gives one the bodily and visual feeling of space and the ability to move freely.

A by-product of Osmond's study was the discovery that people were very resistant to having "their" furniture moved, regardless of whether it was seen as an improvement or not. People have very deep feelings about having their furniture "messed about," as any housewife knows who surprises her family with a new arrangement in the family room.

Furniture is often used to mark our space, our territory which in some sense "belongs" to us and in which we feel comfortable. Patients usually extend into the space surrounding their bed by marking off their territory. Books, magazines, robes, flowers, boxes, makeup will usually be seen lying around instead of neatly tucked away in the drawers and tables the hospital provides. Nonunderstanding by the nursing staff of the purpose of this "clutter" will lead to either a silent war between the nurse and patient in which clutter is put away and magically reappears, or disdain for the patient by the nurse for his or her slovenly habits.

Time

Time, in our culture, is a commodity. We earn it, spend it, save it, waste it, never have enough of it. We refer to time in the same terms as we do money. "Time is money." We recognize that how much time is spent reflects importance.

When someone keeps us waiting it does more to minimize our importance than anything they could possibly say, politely. The very clear message is that what they are doing is more important than anything we could be doing; therefore, they are more important. Schwartz (1974) points out that when we are kept waiting our time is a resource that is ruled solely by the person keeping us waiting. To wait places us in a dependent and subordinate position, which is often acutely felt.

Another communicative aspect of time is duration. Henley (1977) talks about intimate time and impersonal time. An impersonal transaction takes place in 15 minutes or less. Despite how important the transaction may be, the brief period of time gives it an impersonal feel. Intimate transactions happen in extended periods of time—at least thirty minutes or more. The very fact of the extended time for a transaction demands more interaction between the parties which gives the transaction a more personal feel.

I believe that a good deal of the public dissatisfaction with the delivery of medical care of this country is generated by the message sent, but perhaps not intended, by keeping people waiting a long time to see the doctor and then spending a brief amount of time in his or her presence.

Status affects time in much the same way it affects space. The more status one has the less one has to wait. The reasoning, if it were ever verbalized, goes something like this. If you have high status, the things you do are very important, and obviously time cannot be wasted on waiting. The less status you have the less important are the things you do, so you have more time. Actually, we all have only twenty-four hours in a day regardless of our status and probably a very nearly equal number of things to do in that amount of time. As Henley notes, it is a good thing the poor and powerless have more time because they spend so much of it waiting. They wait for nearly every service, in clinics, courts, welfare offices, discount stores, etc. Institutions are like reverse Robin Hoods in that they rob from the poor and give to the rich when it comes to time.

Also like space, time can be invaded by those of higher status on those of lower status. Secretaries, for example, know they must leave the building or else hide to eat their lunch because bosses will interrupt their lunch time to continue their requests for service. Higher status people will interrupt almost any activity or conversation of a lower status person, because they can't wait. The very clear message is a put down and the most common reaction is irritation and resentment.

Sight

Sight seems so natural we seldom realize that we are taught how to "see." For example, although you've probably always suspected it, it is really true that men and women see things differently. Women, in our culture, are expected to play the role of emotional gatekeepers in interpersonal transactions. As a result, they see or attend to different cues or behaviors than men do. They watch faces more than men do, and other small behaviors that are indicators of the emotional state of the speaker.

Eye contact can be so powerful it can seem to have a physical dimension, "He touched me with his eyes." If we catch the eye of another person it demands a different set of behaviors than if we avoid eye contact. We teach children not to look too long at someone who is different, such as the handicapped, because in our culture it is rude. Women know that to catch the eye of a strange man and hold it too long is an invitation to a pickup.

We also touch each other with our eyes for reassurance. If a subordinate is giving a report in the presence of the boss, it is likely you will see him sliding his glance over to the boss checking the okay-ness of his report with the authority. In part, that is why many people do not like to talk on the phone. They cannot see the person's reaction to their message. Occasionally all of us will feel there is something of such import or of such a sensitive nature that it cannot be discussed on the phone. We need to see the impact of the message on the listener to manage the way we say it or the coloring we give it. This is also why people usually get annoyed if someone continues to wear dark glasses while they are conversing. Not only can their eyes and reactions not be seen, but they have an unfair advantage in that they can see the other person's reactions while hiding their own.

There is a strong interaction between sight and speech. Kendon (1967) found that eye contact is one way we monitor taking turns speaking during a conversation. He found one looks away a few seconds before finishing what one has to say, then looks back at the listener just as one stops. This interested gaze while silent invites the other person to speak.

If you never look at the person to whom you are speaking, the listener is made uncomfortable and reads that behavior to mean you are uninterested either in what you are saying, in the listener, or both. People are made equally uncomfortable, however, if you look at them steadily and don't speak. Exline (1974) notes that all primates and perhaps man as well respond to a steady stare without speech as a hostile threat. Generally we read eye contact during speech as self-confidence on the part of the speaker and interest in the listener. Lack of eye contact or a shifting gaze while speaking is generally read as lack of self-confidence or lying. Salesman are specifically trained to maintain eye contact, both to communicate self-confidence and avoid the impression of lying. Actually the folk myth that liars can't look you in the eye does not hold up, although Exline (1974) has some evidence that women have less eye contact when reporting false information than when reporting true information.

Touch

Touch is a basic human need and a powerful method of communication. And like any powerful factor society seeks to control it. One of the first things that children are taught is not to touch. Don't touch others, don't touch their possessions, and certainly don't touch yourself. Years ago children in kindergarten and first grade were graded on a category on their report card headed "Keeps hands to self." In our culture we subordinate tactile communication to visual and verbal communication.

Touch is so powerful that down through the ages it has been attributed the power of healing. The king's touch of medieval times was thought to cure leprosy. Healing by laying of hands has always been a part of certain religious beliefs and is also involved in the approach called holistic medicine. Touching is a unique part of the practice of medicine, and in medical education faculty often speak of the students' need to have a "hands on experience." Agulera (1974) conducted a study and found that when nurses were instructed to touch their patients more frequently than was strictly necessary, the patients talked more and had more positive attitudes towards the nurses.

Somehow, in our culture touching has become associated primarily with sexual behavior, and the belief has evolved that touching takes place in only intimate, personal encounters. Whereas, in fact, a great deal of touching occurs in our society that is nonsexual but rather communicates support and/or dominance. If you were to ask someone "who touches more in our society, men or women?" chances are the response would be women. We tend to think of women kissing each other in greeting or leave-taking and of men as afraid of being thought homosexual if they touch another man. Actually men touch each other a great deal more than women touch each other. For example, men invariably shake hands; team members engage in a good deal of fanny patting or arms around the shoulders. Watch in any office setting and you will see men touch each other in casual ways far more than the women will touch each other.

Touch expresses dominance and status in much the same way as does time and space. Goffman (1967) has described a "touch system" in hospitals where doctors touch nurses, but nurses do not touch doctors. Generally persons touch peers and people of lower status. There is something "wrong" about a person touching someone of higher status. Touching usually goes from the powerful to the less powerful so that older people touch younger people more than vice versa, men touch women more than the reverse, policeman more than suspect, minister more than parishioner, and so forth.

Another dimension of touch is activity or potency. A survey Henley (1977) conducted found that a person was more likely to touch another if they were giving information, advice, or an order, asking a favor or trying to persuade, and less likely to touch when in the more passive role, such as asking for information or advice or being solicited or persuaded.

Touching, like space is also determined by cultural norms. The American and British cultures are far less touch oriented than other cultures. Jourard (1966) counted the number of touches that occurred between a couple in one hour's time. In the various cities he investigated he obtained the following results: San Juan, Puerto Rico, 180; Paris, 110; Gainesville, Florida, 2; London, 0.

Goffman (1967) notes that social class membership also affects touch. He found upper and middle class Britons to hold American-like taboos against physical touch. But as he investigated the lower class rural areas he found body contact during meals and other social occasions quite accepted and normal. However, social class may also reflect a dominance pattern.

In American culture with its basic taboo on touch, touch can express either intimacy or dominance or both. But in casual, nonintimate situations and relationships touch is much more likely to reflect dominance patterns than affection.

Gestures or Body Language

We all are aware of how difficult it is to achieve clear communication. Words mean different things to different people. We don't always listen well. It is easy to misunderstand a perfectly simple sentence. To a large extent we depend on redundancy to clarify our communications. We say the same things over, or say them again in different ways. Another form of redundancy is to communicate the same message with our gestures or body language as the verbal message. When this happens there is congruence in the message being sent verbally and nonverbally and the message is more apt to be received accurately. When these two channels are incongruent, that is, when the nonverbals do not support or send the same as the verbal message, the listener is uneasy, puzzled, or perceives the speaker as lying. Whenever there in incongruence, the listener tends to believe the nonverbal rather than the verbal message. "Actions speak louder than words." The belief seems to be that the nonverbal aspects of communication are less under the speaker's conscious control and therefore more accurately reflect what is really meant or felt.

Many large units of behavior are strictly patterned and carry the primary message, as in for example, courtship behavior. Different cultures have different sequences of interactions and touch that led up to mating. In our culture handholding is early in our courtship pattern, followed by an arm around the shoulders or body, followed by kissing, followed by more body contact, etc. When this pattern is run in the sequence that is known to both parties, communication is clear and both parties understand what is happening. Women sometimes speak of men as being "fast workers." What that usually means is that the fellow has skipped or omitted one or more steps in the courtship sequence taking his partner by surprise. If he follows the proper sequence, no matter how rapidly he may go through them, he is not perceived as "fast."

Scheflen (1965) tells an amusing story of a misunderstanding between English women and Amerian men during World War II when the American Army was stationed in England. American men were amazed at how easy English women were sexually. English women were annoyed at how fast the American men were sexually.

As it turned out, while kissing occurred early in the American courtship stages where events were still under negotiation, so to speak, kissing occurred late in the English courtship pattern and indicated commitment. This one small difference lead to a great deal of misunderstanding and unpleasantness.

Scheflen describes body language that he calls "quasi-courtship behaviors." Quasi-courtship behaviors express alertness, interest, and attractiveness. Some of the elements are what Scheflen calls "preening" behavior. Women may stroke or play with their hair, fix their makeup, rearrange their clothing. Men may stroke their hair, button or adjust their coats, pull up their socks or adjust their tie. Scheflen noted these behaviors appeared not only between lovers, but in various settings where clearly they were in no way intended to be actually sexual in intent. Therefore, they served some monitoring or other function. Two situations were noted in which these quasi-courtship behaviors most often occurred. One was when a member of a group lost interest, withdrew, or was abstracted or excluded. At some point other members would display quasi-courtship behaviors to call the member back to the group. A second circumstance is when one person behaves in a manner that another person feels is inappropriate to their sex role. As when, for example, a woman acts in an aggressive or dominant way, a man may react with quasi-courtship behavior. In this case it seems to act in a gender affirming manner, establishing the masculinity of the male and inviting the female to behave appropriately feminine. These large units of patterned behavior not only transmit a message, but also inform the listener how to respond to the sender.

Illness behaviors are also learned patterns used to communicate the messge "I am ill and should be treated as an ill person." Although the actual physical disorder may be the same for any two people, how they express the fact of their illness may differ greatly. Birdwhistell (1970) in an article entitled "The Expression of Illness in Two American Sub-Cultures" describes the difference in two communities he named Dry Ridge and Green Valley. Although only 15 miles apart in the Kentucky hills they had very different cultures. Dry Ridge valued individualism and had puritanical norms. If one was ill, one was not supposed to talk about it. Illness was a private matter. Illness was to be born with a stiff upper lip. One did not go to a doctor lightly, rather one was forced to go to a doctor. Likewise, medicine was avoided and one did not take to bed unless in extremes.

Illness was communicated in subtle, but for that community, very obvious signs. The skin of the forehead was tightened and smiling reduced. The upper torso was kept hyper-erect with increased "foot planting." Arm and hand movements were slowed with increased precision in gross movement. This stiff upper lip stance is almost an exaggeration or caricature of normal behavior and looks much like anger. If that behavior did not elicit the proper response from kin and associates, the ill person could add the "sag" where the body slumps. The sag could not last too long (only three to five seconds in duration), and the sag and pull together could not occur too frequently (about once in fifteen minutes), or else one was suspected of malingering. Females and the very old or very young could engage in this sag behavior more frequently than could males.

Green Valley was an entirely different community. It was closer knit, more communal, and health concerns were a part of establishing interdependent relationships. Ill health was a public affair, frequently discussed and "enjoyed." Sickness was met with group diagnosis and comparison of symptoms. The norms demanded that the viewer initiate the verbal discussion of the actor's illness.

The actor conveyed illness by compressing the brows, letting the eyelids and upper cheek sag, and letting the lower lip fall slightly away from the teeth. The neck was kept out of tonus, often with a forward or forward and lateral thrust. The upper torso sagged and the belly might be presented. The arms and hands move slowly and the feet drag. Once the illness has been noted and commented on the actor becomes more active with much verbal description and touching, pointing, and rubbing the afflicted parts.

Birdwhistell notes with no comment that the Dry Ridge community has produced four physicians and Green Valley only one.

Generally, Dry Ridge and Green Valley expression of illness might also be characterized as masculine and feminine. Since women in our society are trained to be more comfortable with expression of feeling and dependency than males, they are generally more likely to go to a doctor and overtly and expressively describe their pain and discomfort. Men are more likely to appear at the doctors protesting they came to please their wife and to minimize their pain and discomfort. Since most physicians are men they often discount female complaints, viewing them from their norms as overdone, exaggerated, or "hysterical," often to the disadvantage of their female patients.

An interesting aspect of nonverbal communication is how quickly and accurately people recognize and respond to it when they share the same norms. Rosenthal (1974) and his colleagues investigated the ability of people to accurately recognize an emotion portrayed by an actress in a known content. To the investigators surprise, accuracy was so high that time and time again they cut the exposure time for the people to view the portrayal. Even at 1/24th of a second people were accurate in their identification two-thirds of the time. Another way of recognizing the rapidity of the receiving of nonverbal messages is how quickly people label divergency from their own nonverbal norms as pathology.

Hopefully, this brief description of only a few aspects of nonverbal behavior has increased awareness of this important aspect in interpersonal communications and broadened tolerance for what appears to be deviant interpersonal behavior. Unfortunately, the most usual reaction to a nonverbal impression is a judgmental decision good/bad. Keep in mind that all behaviors must be interpreted in context. Watch for some of the behaviors described in this chapter and see if they are true in your own experience. If not, why not? Look at the situation and the circumstances and try to describe what you see rather than simply label it. Attention to and observation of nonverbal behaviors and the surrounding circumstances will increase your understanding and accuracy. With awareness, curiosity, and an open mind people may remark on your sensitivity, perceptiveness, and clinical intuition.

REFERENCES

Agulera, D. C. Relationships between physical contact and verbal interactions between nurses and patients. *Journal of Psychiatric Nursing*, 5, 5-21, 1967.

Birdwhistell, R. L. *Kinesics and Context: Essays on Body Motion and Communication*. Philadelphia: University of Pennsylvania Press, 1970.

Exline, R. V. Visual interaction: The glances of power and preference. In S. Weitz (Ed.), *Nonverbal Communication*. New York: Oxford University Press, 1974.

Goffman, E. *The Nature of Deference and Demeanor. Interaction Ritual*. Garden City, New York: Doubleday & Co., Inc., 1967.

Goffman, E. *Encounters*. New York: Bobbs-Merrill Co., Inc., 1971.

Hall, E. T. *The Hidden Dimension*. Garden City, New York: Doubleday & Co., Inc., 1969.

Henley, N. M. *Body Politics*. Englewood Cliffs, New Jersey: Prentice-Hall, Inc., 1977.

Jourard, S. M. An exploratory study of body accessibility. *British Journal of Social and Clinical Psychology*, 5, 221-231, 1966.

Kendon, A. Some functions of gaze direction in social interaction. *Acta Psychologica*, 26, 22-63, 1967.

Kleck, R. Physical stigma and task oriented interaction. *Human Relations*, 22, 51-60, 1969.

Osmond, H. The relationship between architect and psychiatrist. In C. Goshen (Ed.), *Psychiatric Architecture*. Washington, D. C.: American Psychiatric Association, 1959.

Rosenthal, R. Body talk and tone of voice: The language without words. *Psychology Today*, 8, 64-68, 1974.

Scheflen, A. E. Quasi-courtship behavior in psychotherapy. *Psychiatry*, 28, 245-247, 1965.

Schwartz, B. Waiting, exchange and power: The distribution of time in social systems. *American Journal of Sociology*, 79, 841-870, 1974.

White, A. G. The patient sits down: A clinical note. *Psychosomatic Medicine*, 15, 236-247, 1953.

Chapter 8

COMMUNICATING WITHIN THE FRAMEWORK OF THE MEDICAL RECORD: NEED TO KNOW VERSUS NICE TO KNOW

Nora P. Kerr

The patient's medical record is generally accepted as a valid monitor of quality of care. We measure quality of care by monitoring patient outcomes as documented in the medical record. We need to know that the patient has achieved the desired outcome: that his physical, nonphysical, and emotional needs have been met.

In the not too distant past, we monitored the creativity, tolerance, and cheerfulness of the caregivers. This is nice to know but certainly is no valid measure of quality of care.

Generally, the patient lacks the knowledge to determine his needs for health services or to make judgments about the quality or benefits of such services. We review the patient record by using criteria that recognize that the acute care hospital provides services needed to:

(1) Protect the patient from adverse effects of the environment.
(2) Prevent complications due to disease or diagnostic or therapeutic maneuvers.
(3) Determine the extent, cause, and progress of the disease or condition.
(4) Provide controlled definitive therapy to halt or reverse the extension of the disease or condition.
(5) Alleviate pain and suffering.

To determine the patient care services best provided in the hospital, we should monitor the record using one of several general criteria:

(1) Skilled observation, vital sign monitoring, use of electronic monitoring devices, etc.
(2) Use of equipment or facilities available only in the hospital.
(3) Preoperative preparation.
(4) Skilled postoperative observation and management.
(5) External pulmonary, circulatory, hepatic, or renal assistance.
(6) Intravenous medication, hyperalimentation, fluid and electrolyte replacement, transfusion, and blood component therapy.
(7) Initial regulation of long-term drug regimes such as anticoagulant therapy, insulin therapy, etc.
(8) Reverse isolation.

The fact that any or all of the above are used is only presumptive evidence of appropriateness. We should also find objective evidence in the medical record that demonstrates the need for those services.

Although in theory the medical record focusing on patient care should be a neutral zone for communication among all health professionals, in practice it is not. Inherent in any discussion of patient care is professional practice. None of the health care disciplines are neutral about that! On those occasions when professionals are not in agreement, the medical record can become a battleground on which is waged a war of professional opinions.

Lack of time for discussion and communication barriers between the health care professions add to the difficulty of communicating within the framework of the medical record. The key to establishing worthwhile records as a measure of quality assurance becomes apparent—establish communication!

Nurses have always been genuinely concerned about continually evaluating and improving the quality of patient care provided. For years, most nursing departments have been evaluating patient care by the audit of nursing records. They have monitored the many aspects of bedside nursing, i.e. the general condition of the patient, the patient's environment, patient safety factors, and so on. They have reviewed charts to determine the completeness and accuracy of nursing notations. Many nursing departments had written standards of care years prior to the present emphasis on quality assurance.

Considering the commitment that nurses have made to evaluate patient care, it is not surprising that the nursing profession is assuming a leadership role in the new emphasis on quality assessment and professional accountability monitored in the medical record.

Medical records reflect the quality of care rendered to patients and therefore play a large role in assessing their care. Positive communication is enhanced when all members of the health care team strive to understand communication conflicts and learn to distinguish basic patterns in professional communication. While technical language serves a useful function when it describes data more precisely and tersely, it is of no use at all when that language is not understood by other professionals who must make use of the information. It is incumbent on each professional to employ technical language only when it clarifies and to avoid it when it obfuscates. But, it is also incumbent on all health care workers to learn the technical language that best communicates relevant information for their understanding of the patient.

Emphasis on practice issues is an important aspect of medical records. The focus of the record should be patient outcome. Methods have been developed for measurement of patient care quality by identification of outcome objectives, analysis of achievement of those objectives, and identification of factors which prevent that outcome.

Health care professionals who focus on quality assurance encounter many questions about the quality of patient care as monitored in the medical record.

(1) Who is the coordinator of patient care? Who assigns responsibilities?
(2) Is this assignment of responsibility the function of the physician? The nurse? The administration?
(3) Can the role of all members of the health care team in arriving at actual patient care outcomes be identified?

These questions can be answered when all members of the health care team work cooperatively to the advantage of the patient.

For instance, a patient admitted with uncontrolled diabetes should have his blood sugar controlled at discharge—this is the desired outcome. This will be influenced by serveral members of

the health care team, each of whom has distinct responsibilities.
   (1) Prescription of the type and amount of insulin and diet and overall direction of therapy are physician responsibilities.
   (2) Administration of insulin, educating the patient in insulin self-administration, and compliance with dietary restrictions are within the realm of nursing.
   (3) Diet instructions are under the guidance of the dietician.
   (4) Laboratory personnel are responsible for collecting the blood and interpreting the results.
   (5) Physical Therapy may be asked to instruct the patient in proper methods of daily exercise.
   (6) The Social Service Department may be called upon to assist the patient in locating community and agency services available to him.

The patient's achievement of the desired outcome, his knowledge, and how his therapy is directed and coordinated is the result of many health care professionals cooperating, each within his own area of competency, to provide the desired patient outcome.

The record should be viewed as a patient record rather than a medical record. By organizing all of the problems of the patient, the patient record can become the tool for measuring the quality and comprehensiveness of care. The patient record should be the tool for continuous coordination of the patient's care among the members of the health care team. Each health care professional should make his or her observations and recommendations on the same record to document the contribution of all members of the health care team. This will provide for checks and balances in the care of the patient, giving the patient the advantage of the best quality of care.

Prerequisites to communication among the members of the health care professions are recognition and respect for the unique contribution of each member of the health care team. Unfortunately, many hospitals include a few persons who never develop respect for the contribution of others. Too often, important information in the medical record is overlooked by professionals who regard as relevant only those portions of the record contributed by members of their own profession. Awareness that patient care represents a blending of more than one professional discipline and that health care providers are accountable for their activities leads to effective communication among the members of the health care team.

No member of the health care team need feel threatened by a quality assurance program whose focus is improved quality of care. Focusing on the patient can unite the efforts of all health care professionals. It is the responsibility of each health care discipline to respond to the deficiencies, each to his own profession.

Failure to assign accountability for practice deficiencies may destroy a viable educational tool—the medical record. It may negate positive improvements in patient care and hamper effective communication among the members of the health care team.

REFERENCES

Davis, F. (Ed.). *The Nursing Profession*. New York: John Wiley & Sons, Inc., 1966.

Friedson, E. *Professional Dominance: Social Structure of Medical Care*. New York: Atherton Press, 1970.

Marble, A., White, P., Bradley, R. F., and Krall, L. P. (Eds.). *Joslin's Diabetes Mellitus*. Philadelphia: Lea & Febiger, 1971.

Mayers, M. G. Program evaluation in community health nursing: A search for assessment criteria. *Nursing Outlook, 20,* 323-326, 1972.

Weeds, L. *Medical Records, Medical Education and Patient Care*. Cleveland: Case Western Reserve University Press, 1969.

Chapter 9

WHO SAID COMMUNICATION WAS EASY?
OR
REBUILDING THE TITANIC

Lowell F. Bernard

The critical force in the development of any program to enhance communication is that of assembling the most effective team to research, design and implement it. At first glance that may seem obvious but is it really? A historical example may help elucidate some of the problems involved.

Remember the Titanic? Constructed in England in the late 1920s, it was considered to be the ultimate in shipbuilding design and construction. It was called "unsinkable" by those who built it. The finest staff of engineers and shipbuilders had scrutinized every detail. Indeed, the Titanic was believed to be the safest ship afloat. Yet, the tragic events of her maiden voyage are all too familiar today.

What might have been some of the factors behind the demise of the Titanic? Was it a failure of communication among the staff? Was it a false sense of security ensuing from the construction team's publicity prior to the voyage? Or was it a failure on the part of the crew to exercise reasonable caution in dangerous waters? It was probably a combination of these and other factors that placed the ship in its ultimate peril. A rehabilitation program has the potential to float or sink as a function of similar factors.

Each of the Titanic's passengers had dreams and expectations for the voyage and what lay beyond when they reached their destination. As the few survivors were plucked from the dark, frigid waters of the North Atlantic, the crushing pain and emotional devastation of this experience must have been clearly visible. They had lived through the sinking of the "unsinkable" Titanic. Their faces and comments probably reflected a loss of confidence in anything they might be told. The real tragedy of the Titanic, then, may lie in the fact that each passenger was the victim of a credibility gap in communication.

Patients, like the Titanic passengers, have had their goals and dreams prematurely snatched from them. It is the health care professional's challenge to help them build a future life based upon realizable goals, recognizing their limitations. It is imperative that, on the voyage to the realization of those goals, communication breakdowns, unrealistic expectations and a lack of caution do not shipwreck their rehabilitation program. At this juncture, one cannot separate the ship from its passengers any more than one can separate the psyche from the soma of the patient.

What is the best way to rebuild our patients' new lives? Health care professionals must explore a variety of ways that members might more effectively implement their skills. To gain maximum efficiency, a total team plan must evolve in which every member is sufficiently informed to be effectively used from the beginning to the end of the program. Further, false hopes must not be generated and reasonable caution must be exercised when embarking on new approaches.

Imagine that the Titanic is to be rebuilt using all the information learned from the prior tragedy and from similar, more recent events. Can we develop a vessel that is unsinkable? The thought of such a challenge staggers the imagination. Is such a venture realistic? What would be required to meet the goal; what would be the financial cost? Who should comprise the team that would make it a reality? Like the engineers and shipbuilders who might be called upon to rebuild the Titanic, health care professionals are confronted with the task of preventing health-care related disasters caused by communication gaps with patients who have had a devastating experience in their lives. In a sense, health care professionals have been called upon to "rebuild the Titanic . . ." to rehabilitate its survivors and to prevent new victims.

Who are the individuals that constitute an ideal rehabilitation team? The physician, dentist, nurse, social worker, patient, patient's family, health educator, and the list goes on. Where it stops depends largely on the scope of the program being planned. However, if such varied members are to be included in a team, it is clear that problems of education and communication will arise. In part, for this reason, there is a growing recognition that a competent health educator is needed to complement the health care team. The health educator brings with him a specialized knowledge of how to develop effective communication techniques.

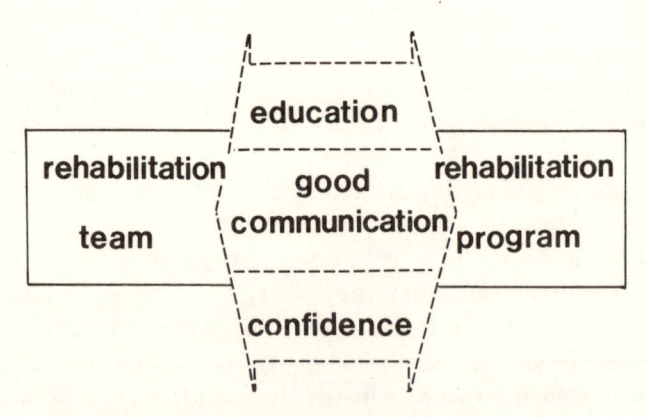

Figure 9-1. Interface of elements of communication in rehabilitation programs.

Remember, the Titanic ran into difficulty when communication among its crew became confused or misinterpreted. Similarly, all members of the rehabilitation team, but especially the patient, must clearly understand why various courses of action have been prescribed as part of his or her rehabilitation program; otherwise, confusion, misinterpretation, lack of behavior change and other failures may result. The consequences, of course, will be evident in the lack of confidence patients exhibit in members of the team, slow recovery, misuse of rehabilitation systems and, ultimately, higher costs for treatment as more professional time is required for each patient. The omission of any member of the team during the rehabilitation process is an invitation to disaster for the patient.

Construction of a health care or rehabilitation team which includes the patient as a member does offer some hope for an "unsinkable" ship. This represents the current "ultimate" in health care program design. As with rebuilding the Titanic, there are several factors that may enhance or detract from even the most effective team efforts, i.e. may cause the ship to float or sink. For example, the interacting group should be kept as small as is functionally possible. Time and financial accountability must be considered. It is more important that all team members have mutual respect for the qualities that each brings to the program.

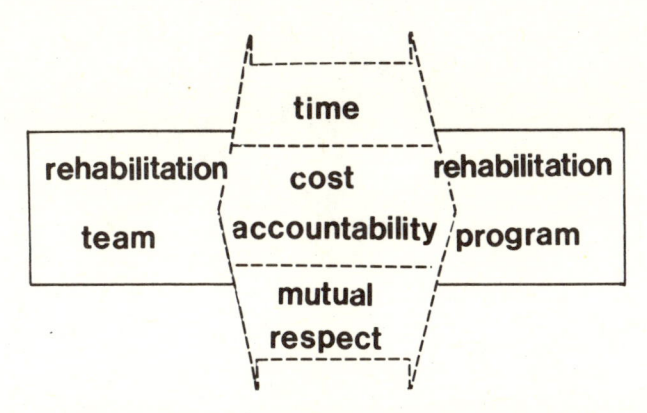

Figure 9-2. Factors that may effect the team effort.

In addition to professional knowledge, each member brings his or her educational background and his or her personal beliefs and prejudices. However, since it is the patient whose program is being planned and whose goals are to be realized, a good health care team will explore each delicate issue. They will weigh all decisions regarding program direction in light of how attitudes and beliefs will affect the motivation of team members in reaching their goal or objective.

In addition, a knowledge and respect for each person's background will permit messages geared to the understanding level of all of the participants of the team. We have been highly trained and it is difficult to filter the necessary, basic information and concentrate it into a message with meaning . The question in the past was, just how much information is needed by the patient. Today, the question is, just how can we most effectively convey the information to the patient. In general, the team must be sensitive to the varied and individual needs of the patient, and these needs are far from static throughout the patient's life.

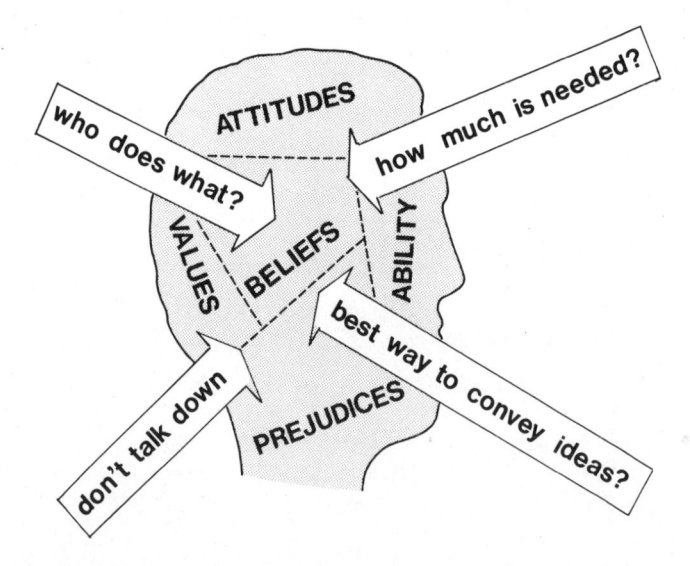

Figure 9-3. Multifaceted considerations in the communication process.

The concerns mentioned previously are issues for every member of a rehabilitation team as it prepares program plans with the patient. They may not represent all the considerations, but to overlook any of these concerns can be likened to going into a poker game with an incomplete deck of cards. The team will have greatly altered its chances of success in producing winning hands.

Up to this point we have considered the factors that contribute to a more effective planning team. What about the actual techniques of communicating among members of the team? This is one of the points at which the health educator can provide useful contributions.

Many experiments have been undertaken to determine how people learn. Each has shown that well-selected audiovisual aids enhance the speed and accuracy of communication between instructor and recipient. In recent years a shift has occurred in education which has resulted in a move away from the "teacher centered" lecture style to a "recipient-centered," self-learning style.

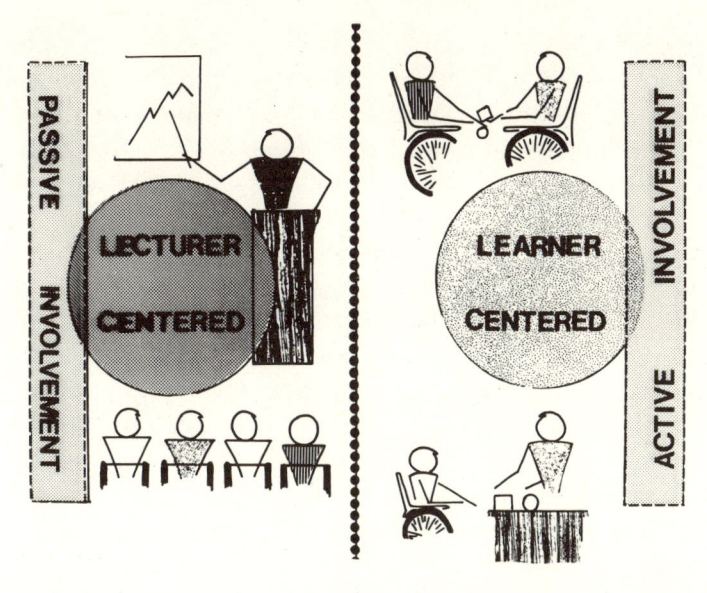

Figure 9-4. In recent years a shift has occurred in education which has resulted in a move from the "teacher centered" lecture style to a "recipient-centered," self-learning style.

The latter is a greater challenge for all because it shifts the burden of instruction from the educator and assumes that recipients will be motivated to learn on their own. This means that the professional team member acts as a facilitator of the learning experience. It requires patience and a good set of educational objectives to produce an environment conducive to individual learning. The patient, in the health care setting, sets his or her own pace and the professional is available to guide or answer questions from the patient and family. Although some professionals may find it difficult to relinquish their leadership role because they feel it diminishes their professional responsibility, it is hoped that most professionals will accept the challenge to allow the patient this exciting new freedom in learning. It can provide an atmosphere of positive motivation and modification of behavior in the direction of assuming greater responsibility for self. This is not to say that the professional need not be available to guide the patients if they stray from the desired path. This approach permits the professional more time to work with greater numbers of patients and their families who are also in need of his or her expertise. It also provides time that can be used to develop ever improving rehabilitation plans for patients and to assist in the selection and/or creation of audiovisual aids that will enhance those plans.

Audiovisual aids can put difficult concepts into a form of easily understood communication. They offer the opportunity to provide a common basis for understanding through the presentation of a uniform message. Audiovisual aids, if effectively developed or selected, can enhance and reinforce the professionals' program with the patient and the patient's family. They can assist the professional in overcoming the space-time barrier of words alone by capturing action at one critical time in an event and calling it back for future "replay." Audiovisual aids permit reexamination of an explanation as often as is necessary for the patient or family to comprehend.

What audiovisual aids cannot do, however, is guarantee positive motivation or behavioral modification.

With the assistance of audiovisual aids, patients are able to "enter" the body in order to see how it works normally and to see how it functions as it has been altered by disease, injury, or medical-surgical techniques. Or a patient can examine prosthetic devices at work before and after they are placed in the body. Such a capacity to see and hear offers the opportunity for greater comprehension.

Visual aids may be used to increase the impact of a program: to increase and make uniform the understanding among team members, to insure consistent expectations, and to provide information most effectively and efficiently. How and when each visual aid might be used should rest with the entire rehabilitation team.

Before describing the strengths and weaknesses of several audiovisual techniques, a few general pitfalls must be mentioned. There is a tendency on the part of some professionals to over-use audiovisual aids. At other times, professionals may initially incorporate poorly planned aids as supplements to their program because such aids are readily available and offer the "path of least resistance." Still other professionals fall innocently into the trap of

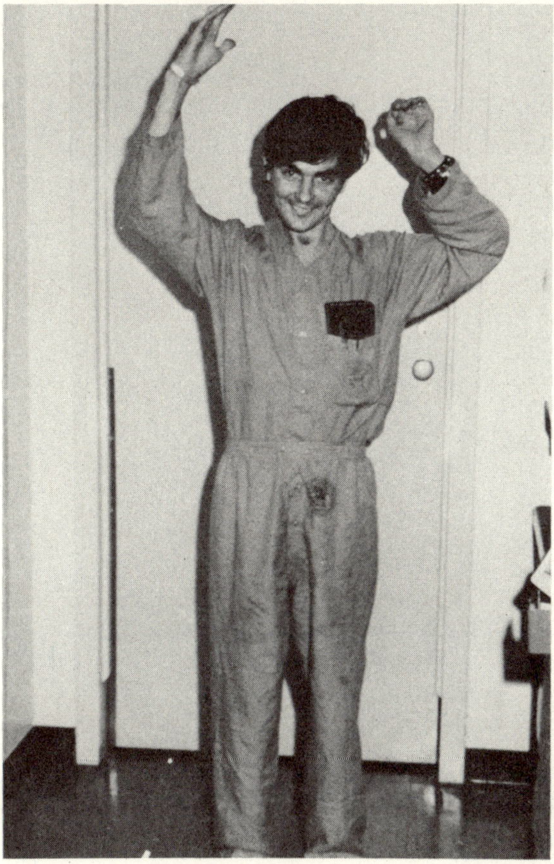

Figure 9-5. Audiovisual aids can capture action at one critical time in an event and call it back for future replay, for example, this photograph captures a patient standing unassisted for the first time.

attempting to include too much in their message with the result that the recipient becomes confused, mentally fatigued, or turned-off. The ultimate results, of course, are negative in that the patients misunderstand the information or modify their behavior incorrectly. The lesson to be learned from this consequence is: audiovisual aids should be carefully selected. If the correct material does not

120　　　　　　*Communications In A Health Care Setting*

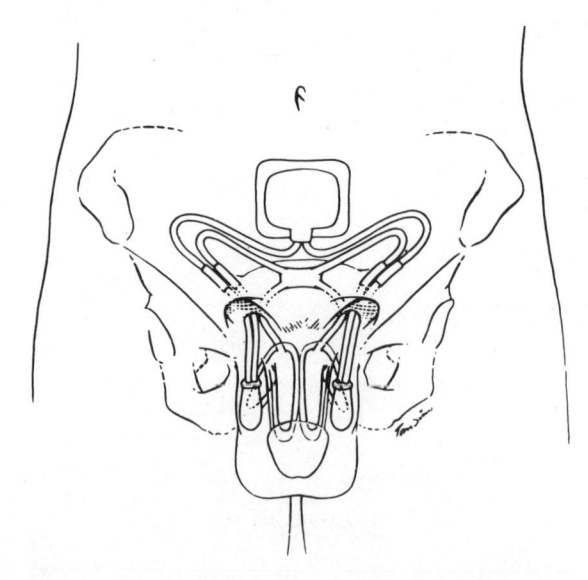

Figure 9-6. Patients are able to enter the body to see how it works, for example, how a surgically implanted penile prosthesis functions.

EFFECTIVE VISUALS ?

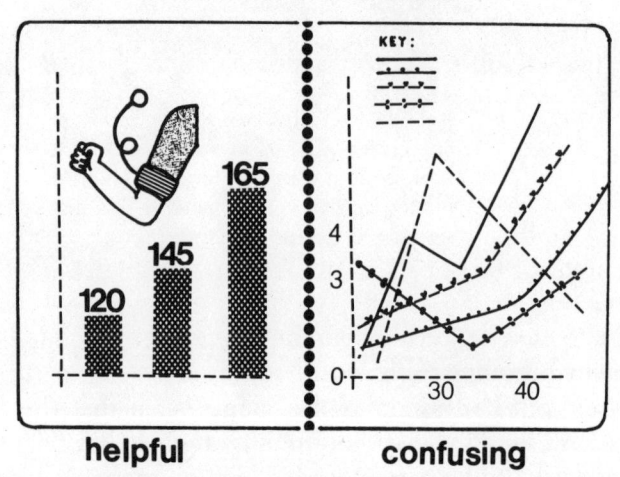

helpful　　　　　　**confusing**

Figure 9-7. Examples of helpful and confusing visual aids.

exist or is not available, the professional has an obligation to help create it.

Selection of Audiovisual Aids

Thirty-Five mm slides permit maximum flexibility in program presentation. As new information becomes available, new slides can be prepared and inserted into a program at little expense. Outdated material can be removed without destroying the entire program. This feature, ease of editing, along with relatively low cost, makes slides an ideal visual starting point in any program development. As with all visual aids, slides should have a clear focal point, be attractive in color, bold, and simple. A good rule of thumb is to have only the first point on the screen as that point is being discussed, then progressively add other points with additional slides and, finally, have all points listed on the final slide to provide a summary. Salient facts may be reemphasized by having one or more slides repeated in the program.

Uniform verbal presentations can be presented with slides in a variety of ways. The best method, of course, is to use a system which inserts inaudible signals on a pretaped sound track that activates the progress of the slides in the projector. Smooth presentations can be presented by using two slide projectors working off a dissolve unit that is activated by a synchronizing tape record-playback unit. This prevents the jerking sensation that accompanies the use of a single projector system as the slides are projected on the screen.

A number of companies have begun preparing filmstrips in which the visuals are attached in a preselected sequence that cannot be altered. The advantage of this method is in the production of multiple units for mass distribution. The programs sometimes come in cartridges for ease in storage and use in specially designed projectors. This permits individuals who are not trained in the use of audiovisual equipment to preview shows without staff assistance. In some cases equipment contains sound systems that permit simultaneous use of audiotapes with the narrative to supplement the visuals. Special "programmed-learning" multimedia modules have been developed using this format combined with written material

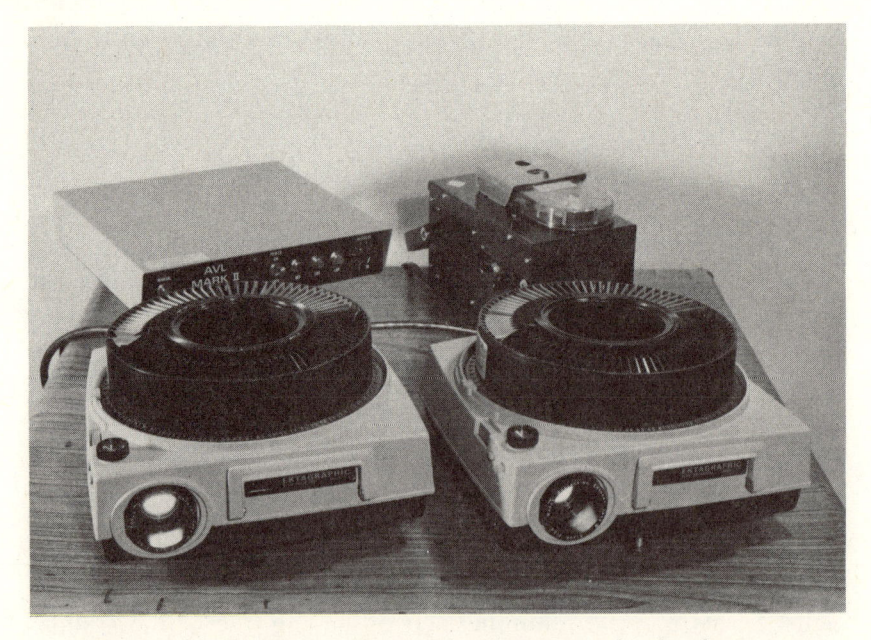

Figure 9-8. Illustrations of two slide projectors and a dissolve unit.

that assists the viewer in pacing his or her learning. Through written questions the recipient can determine whether key points have been learned. Unfortunately, these programs do not have follow-up components to determine if the information has led to any modification of behavior. More evaluation work is required to determine the effectiveness of this format.

The most resorted to modality in the communication arts is the film. Its strength lies in its ability to depict motion of objects better than any other visual form, except for actual live demonstrations of the object by a competent professional. Films come in two size formats, 8mm and 16mm. The former is usually placed in what is called a continuous loop cartridge so that it does not have to be rewound after a showing. Although these films occasionally jam in the cartridge, get badly scratched, have flaking of the sound track, or wear out and tear, drawbacks which should be considered, the cartridges nonetheless permit inexperienced people to show the films. These projectors have been designed to permit viewing films in relatively small rooms. This capability has special meaning where space is at a premium, and there is not sufficient staff required to handle the more complex 16mm movie projector.

One problem with films is that they are very expensive to produce, especially if they have animated sequences. Such films, once purchased, tend to be used to justify their high cost, even when portions become outdated. A better use for these films would be the development of single concept "filmettes," a term I coined when I took sections cut from existing films that served a specific educational purpose and used these sections in various combinations to supplement a presentation. Animation sections may be lifted out of a technical film designed as a Career Training film. The intent of the "filmette" can thus be varied by the person using it. It can demonstrate how cells form tissues and how tissues basically function in the body. It can be used to explain how cancer spreads or how it can be detected by examining exfoliated cells. The value of this modality lies not only in its ability to build on the motion achieved through animation, but that the shortened length permits the "filmette" to supplement rather than usurp the professional. By eliminating the prepared film sound track, professionals can use any number of different scripts to explain the phenomenon being demonstrated.

A professional does not have to discard an expensive film that has outdated or incorrect information. Simply by cutting these sections out, one can redefine the use of the remaining portions of the film.

Overhead transparencies have been used for many years in the classroom. They offer convenience at a low cost and can quickly be prepared. There are, however, some simple rules to follow in the preparation of effective overhead transparencies. The first and most important rule holds true for all visual aids: make the message as simple as possible. Do not crowd all the needed information on one transparency. Design it carefully so that it permits a gradual unfolding of the story. In the case of overhead transparencies, this can be accomplished by a technique called "barn-dooring," which is accomplished by placing an opaque sheet over portions of the transparency that you do not yet wish to expose to the audience. The barn door may contain an outline of key information you may wish to convey. It helps create a relaxed, well-organized presentation.

Models or specimens may also be useful to include in a

multimedia presentation. They are especially helpful if part of the program calls for the patient, or the patient's family, to learn how to use equipment, prostheses, or techniques. To heighten the educational impact a slide-tape show or filmette may be used as a supplement. People learn more by becoming directly involved, and functional models can greatly increase their involvement in the total learning experience.

Television in recent years has grown by use of the portable closed-circuit equipment, which allows taping activities and immediately replaying them for reexamination and discussion. It is an effective technique for short-term evaluation, long-term reevaluation, or comparison activities. Although the basic videotape equipment is more costly than other techniques mentioned, it does open up new possibilities in patient and family education that cannot be handled with the same ease using the other forms of audiovisual aids previously mentioned. A precaution to be remembered when using this equipment: do not make the mistake of using this media in a static form. It is a media of motion and should not contain lengthy presentations of professionals sitting or standing in front of a camera explaining a concept. Exploit the dynamic qualities of the medium. If you have questions about improved use of this technique of communication, seek help from a local television station. Often professional communication staff will provide guidance in program development to insure that television is used properly.

Another communication technique that has recently become financially feasible is that of the minicomputer. With the development of the minicomputer a new educational modality was created. Although largely used by small businesses and industry to maintain inventory control, they also have direct educational applications. If professionals in the health delivery system will recognize the value of computers now they can begin planning educational approaches for the future that will greatly enhance both treatment and rehabilitation modalities of medicine. The minicomputer can offer information on a one-to-one basis in general health education and preventive health maintenance. With proper planning, programs can be developed that will extend the function of the professional rehabilitation team even into the home. The effects of the rehabilitation programs can then be evaluated on a

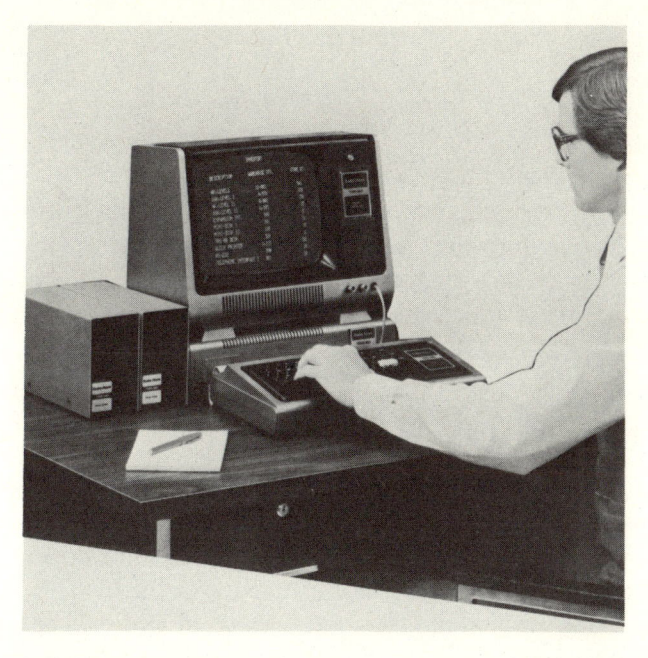

Figure 9-9. The mini-computer is a new educational and communication modality.

daily basis by the patient and the patient's family. Problem areas can be anticipated using minicomputer programs and instructions given that will help the patient prevent, or at least reduce, the possiblity of complications at home.

There are many effective ways of reaching the patient with high quality programs. One does not have to expend large sums of money or use highly exotic equipment in special environments constructed solely for that equipment's use. The key to successful programs lies in the careful selection by a well-rounded rehabilitation team composed of the professionals, the patient, and the patient's family. This team must carefully select from existing materials, or prepare new materials to meet the objectives of their program. In each case the patient and his or her family differ and, thus, require individual attention. The most effective program is the one that states the problem simply, gives a realistic approach, involves the participant in the learning process, and, finally, has some form of follow-up to determine whether the goals of the program have been realized.

Additional Caution

Do not fall victim to the smooth talking salesman who claims to have the latest equipment and insists that it cannot fail to work for you. Check with others in the field. There may be less expensive methods already developed that will accomplish the proposed task. Use the valuable professional resources in the community that are available. Above all, do not be afraid to experiment. Developing an audiovisual program is a challenge well worth your time and effort.

CONCLUSION

Recognizing that the rehabilitation of a patient involves the modification of attitudes and behavior of the patient and those around him, the rehabilitation team must take into consideration all factors that impinge on these attitudes and behavior.

The composition of the rehabilitation team is of primary concern. The team should be well balanced and include a behavioral scientist. The patient and members of the patient's family should be included in the rehabilitation team, and the focus of the resulting program should involve them throughout its implementation.

To be maximally effective, the rehabilitation program should be patient-oriented rather than professional-oriented. Just as in education, a new atmosphere of learning must be developed, one in which the professional acts as a facilitator of learning rather than merely a lecturer. What does this mean in terms of the rehabilitation team? Members must establish an environment conducive to learning. They must react with warmth, understanding, and support; and they must be open to discussion among themselves. The patient must be involved in the design of his or her own rehabilitation module. The activity becomes a self-learning experience for everyone involved.

Any rehabilitation plan can be improved by proper planning. Such careful planning should include the correct selection and use of audiovisual aids at the appropriate time to reinforce or clarify difficult concepts. These aids should be simple, colorful, and dynamic and presented at a pace that will enhance audiovisual learning by the patient. There are many community resources available to the team to assist in the preparation of effective audiovisual aids for this purpose.

In closing, each member of the team must ask themselves which deserves our greater care: the multi-million dollar rebuilding of the Titanic, where a cost-effectiveness analysis can be clearly demonstrated; or the rebuilding and rehabilitation of a patient who has been entrusted to our care? Let us become patient-centered in our treatment modality, rather than self-centered or cost-centered.

We have often heard the quote "talk is cheap" meaning that anyone can speak out on a given subject; however, effective communication is difficult. It takes careful teamwork with a focus on involvement of the entire team. Hopefully some of the ideas presented in this chapter will stimulate readers to become more effective communicators.

SECTION III

Analyzing the special needs and characteristics of patients with a specific illness or disability is an essential first step in anticipating and solving communication problems. Everyone must know what is being communicated by both patients and staff before change can be implemented and communication patterns improved.

Chapters in the following section illustrate how communication problems may be ameliorated or resolved in four discrete areas of medical practice: spinal cord injury, chronic renal failure, pediatric oncology, and chronic pain. As a unit, the chapters highlight the varied approaches that may lead to a better understanding of communication, i.e. focusing on the unique problems of staff members, patients and their families, or on previous coping patterns.

Chapter 10

FACILITATING COMMUNICATION: AN AID TO EFFECTIVE TREATMENT ON THE RENAL DIALYSIS UNIT

Lynne C. Rustad

For victims of the disease and the professionals who treat them, chronic renal failure is among the most emotionally frustrating and challenging of all medical problems. They must cope not only with the problems of chronic illness but often with recurrent acute episodes that can be life-threatening and demoralizing. Unfortunately, some of the devices used by both patients and staff to cope with the threat of the illness and maintain some semblance of emotional equilibrium may disrupt communication, leading to conflict and hindering effective treatment. When conflicts arise and treatment flounders, however, problems are frequently seen as residing primarily or exclusively in the patient, and he or she may be referred to a mental health professional for evaluation and treatment. However, effectiveness of the treatment may be severely limited since only one member of what is actually a disturbed system is receiving treatment and support. Attention to the stresses experienced by both patients and caregivers is necessary. An understanding of these stresses and ways in which communication may be disrupted by individuals' attempts to cope with them can provide a basis for intervening directly in the disturbed system.

In the discussion to follow, stresses experienced by patients and staff and some of the maladaptive devices used for dealing with them will be discussed. Finally, some suggestions will be offered to help professionals cope more effectively so that communication will be facilitated and treatment effectiveness enhanced rather than diminished.

Sources of Stress for the Individual with Chronic Renal Failure

Patients on chronic hemodialysis often feel physically ill. They may experience chronic or intermittent fatigue, lethargy, itching, GI distress, cramps, and sensory loss and pain due to neuropathy. They live with the constant threat of further deterioration and death. Recurrent crises such as blocked or infected fistulas, loss of access routes, hypotensive crises, angina, and amputations are not uncommon. Death or deterioration of other patients on the dialysis unit serve as constant reminders of their own vulnerability. Even patients with effectively functioning kidney transplants do not escape these concerns (Ford & Castelnuovo-Tedesco, 1977). They may live with the constant fear of rejection—even rejection crises—and are well aware that the immunosuppressive agents that help to prevent rejection can leave them relatively defenseless should infection strike.

Renal failure also tends to disrupt the patient's body image, with resultant anxiety and loss of self-esteem. Urination, taken so much for granted in a healthy population, can become an obsession for patients on dialysis who may keep careful records of their daily urine output, being much less concerned about the quality of the urine produced by their kidneys than their ability to maintain this "normal" function. Arms distorted by fistulas may cause some patients to refuse to wear short-sleeved blouses or shirts. Body boundaries may be severely threatened by the necessity of having machines and other people take over the kidneys' normal function of cleansing the blood. Repeated invasion of the body with needles and watching the blood flow outside of the body may further contribute to the patient's fears about the faltering integrity of his body boundaries, as may sensory loss, especially the visual and tactile losses seen in diabetic patients.

Patients must also cope with psychosocial stresses arising from the disease and its treatment. Major modifications in life-style and habits are required. Time is restricted for dialysis patients by the requirement that fifteen or more hours each week be devoted to the dialysis itself and travel to and from the center. Scheduling problems that can add several additional hours to time spent at the center may interfere with vocational, family, and recreational activities. For some patients, home dialysis is a desirable alternative to center-based dialysis, allowing them and their families increased flexibility and control over their care. However, this alternative also calls for greater responsibility and makes considerable demands on the time and emotional and physical energy of family members (Streltzer, Finkelstein, Feigenbaum, Kitsen, & Cohn, 1976).

Among the most frustrating restrictions experienced by the patient are those imposed by the renal diet. Modifying life-long habits to meet stringent restrictions on protein, sodium, potassium, and fluid intake is most difficult. It is the rare patient, indeed, who does not feel deprived by this diet regimen. It is particularly difficult for those patients who, in the past, drank or ate as a means of relieving tension and for those accustomed to a "meat and potatoes" diet. At the same time that food is restricted, the patient is asked to take substantial quantities of a variety of oral medications. Learning about these drugs and complying with a daily therapeutic regimen adds yet another stress.

Role changes brought about by chronic disease and its treatment are disruptive for the family as well as the patient (Carpenter, 1974; Skipper, Fink, & Hallenbeck, 1969). Loss of employment because of illness with consequent loss of the family "breadwinner" role may seriously threaten self-esteem. Financial insecurity and a reduced standard of living can contribute significantly to family conflict, which may actually be worsened if the formerly nonworking member of the couple must seek employment to help alleviate financial distress. Marital relationships may be strained further by changes in sexual activity. Estimates of sexual dysfunction, including impotence, in male renal patients range from 20-80 percent (Czaczkes & Kaplan-Denour, 1978).

Given the numerous stresses discussed above, there remains one final and very important issue to be considered: that of the dependency engendered by chronic hemodialysis (Reichsman & Levy, 1974) and the conflicting demands made on the patient for independence. This situation has been characterized by Alexander (1976) as a "Double-Bind" phenomenon. In order for a double-bind situation to occur, an individual must receive one message overtly while receiving a contradictory message covertly, and there must be no escape from the situation. This would appear to be a very central problem for hemodialysis patients. They are dependent for their life and their well-being on the machine, the staff caring for them, and on the institution which makes this care possible. They are expected to trust their caregivers, obey orders, and not question professional judgement. At the same time, obeying these very orders, e.g. complying with medication and diet regimens, requires considerable independence and discipline. For individuals caught between these conflicting expectations there may appear to be no exit except for the fatal decision to terminate dialysis, a solution not uncommonly entertained by these people.

Sources of Stress for the Dialysis Staff

Having reviewed some major sources of stress for patients, it is now time to consider some of the difficulties experienced by professionals working in the dialysis setting. Underlying a number of these difficulties is the fact that the renal staff is subjected to the stresses involved in the delivery of both acute and chronic care. As do professionals in other acute settings, dialysis personnel must cope with intensive patient contact, emergency procedures, work schedule problems, severe illness, and death. At the same time, however, they must also cope with stresses arising from the close involvement with patients, which is characteristic of the extended care setting. Thus, death of dialysis patients for whom the staff has cared for over a long period of time is more likely to be experienced as a personal loss, and perhaps a personal failure, than would be the case on an acute unit where patients are less well known. The extended and intensive investment of time and energy in care of patients also makes it difficult to accept patient deterioration, which seems to proceed in spite of care, as well as the noncompliance which persists in spite of the staff's best efforts to remedy it.

Dialysis personnel may also find themselves in the unfortunate position of providing a convenient focus for their patients' frustration and anger arising from other sources such as illness or personal or family problems. While this displacement of anger may occur in any setting, it is likely to be more stressful on the unit. Because of the extended patient-staff relationship, patients tend to be well aware of weaknesses and areas of sensitivity in individual staff members and strike at these areas when they are angry. Patient knowledge and understanding of unit personnel also extends to intrastaff conflicts. Although a professional staff without differences of opinion would be most unusual, in the acute setting patients may remain unaware of them. On the dialysis unit, such disagreements may be common knowledge and a topic for discussion among patients. At times, they may even use this information manipulatively to play one staff member against another with resultant escalation of the conflict.

Finally, some staff members must cope with the stress of their own "Double-Bind" phenomenon. Nurses and technicians on the dialysis unit are charged with significant responsibilities that are not usually shared by their colleagues in other settings. In terms of procedures, decision-making, and active involvement in care, they are asked to take on some duties which, in other settings, might be considered the province of medical staff. At times, however, it is expected that they be totally dependent on the judgment and orders of physicians. This role duality can result in confusion, frustration, and even resentment.

Coping with Stress

How people handle psychological and physical stress depends on a number of factors including: (1) their individual anatomical and physiological make-up, (2) how they learned to cope with stress as they matured by observing family members, and (3) the way in which people in their present environment respond to their attempts to handle the stress. While there is a wide range in individual ability to deal with stress, even those with the strongest personalities may encounter situations in which they feel weak, helpless, and unable to cope effectively. Acute and severe chronic illness are two such situations, and staff members as well as patients may find themselves unprepared to react to an appropriate and effective manner (Moos, 1977). Instead, they may respond to the anxiety and depression aroused by illness with a variety of maneuvers which intensify their distress and are effective only in isolating them from others who may be helpful. In the sections to follow, some of the maladaptive coping patterns used by patients and staff members will be discussed.

Patient Coping Devices

Somatic complaints are among the most commonly encountered signs of distress on any medical service and the renal dialysis unit is no exception. While some of the reported symptoms reflect organic disease processes, others appear to be partly or exclusively psychogenic in origin. It is important to keep in mind, however, that, regardless of etiology, these symptoms are usually only too real for the patient. They may reflect anxiety and confusion about, or absorption in, the illness. At other times they represent a call for attention and aid for psychological distress that patients are reluctant to express directly or are not fully aware of themselves. Unfortunately, rather than gaining the attention and help desired, these symptoms often do no more than earn for the patient the label of hypochondriac.

The dependency on staff members and machines discussed earlier may lead patients to the conclusion that they have little, if any, control over their own lives. Feeling helpless and lacking the energy or motivation to fight to maintain control in areas of life where it may be possible, some patients essentially retire and settle for an extemely *passive and dependent adjustment*. Initially, these individuals may be seen as "good patients" on the unit since they tend to be compliant and allow staff members to take over their care without resistance or questioning. However, this dependency is not likely to serve them well outside of the hospital where they must take considerable responsibility for complying with the medication and diet regimen. In addition, the staff (and the patient's family) are likely to tire of this behavior over the course of time and find that whatever initial gratification they derived from the dependency does not compensate for the patient's demanding behavior and lack of responsibility. If staff members respond by withdrawing support, as they may be tempted to do, the patient feels even more vulnerable.

At times, patients use a very different technique to deal with the anxiety engendered by dependency and loss of control. They fight fiercely to protect themselves by *maintaining the appearance of independence*. They may be quite guarded, hoping to keep at least their thoughts and fears private and under their own control. They may also be very suspicious and distrustful of staff members, questioning procedures endlessly and even implying that the professionals treating them are not competent. Noncompliance may be used to show everyone who is really in control. While these tactics may temporarily protect patients, over time distress increases because hidden fears cannot be subjected to reality testing and staff members are alienated by the patient's inaccessibility.

When patients feel overwhelmed by their situation and decide that they are not being heard or that no one could help them even if they were heard, they may respond by *withdrawing*. Such withdrawal may be reflected in the patient's spending increasing amounts of time alone and limiting social contacts and verbal and affective communication. In the extreme, the patient may be virtually mute. Such behavior is most frustrating for professionals, especially if they would like to help the patient. They may respond by giving the patient "pep talks" or by withdrawing, leaving the patient even more lonely, isolated, and helpless.

*Rath*er than withdrawing, some patients are only too vocal in their distress. However, it is not likely to be fear and sadness which are expressed so openly: for patients of either sex, but particularly for men in our culture, the expression of anger is considered to be more socially acceptable. Fear and frustration are reflected in *verbal abusiveness* of staff and other patients, complaints about the quality of care, anger at modifications in their dialysis schedule, and accusations that the staff does not care about them. Unfortunately, this behavior is often taken at face value and anger is met with anger, the staff failing to see that the abusiveness hides other feelings that the patient is afraid to express.

Perhaps no problem on the dialysis unit is more common, more refractory to treatment, and more frustrating for care-givers than *noncompliance*. In part, the magnitude of this problem may reflect that fact that noncompliance is often seen as *a* problem—a unitary phenomenon—when in reality it may be an indirect expression of a number of different problems (Barofsky, 1978). In some cases, noncompliance early in dialysis reflects straightforward misunderstanding or lack of information about diet requirements. Frequently, it is a signal of distress of one kind or another. For some new dialysis patients who feel deprived because they have experienced many losses and have had to make numerous adjustments in life-style, diet restrictions provide the final blow. Too much is expected too soon and they respond by giving up attempts to comply. For others, noncompliance with regimen may reflect a denial of the disease. They are acting "as if" the disease does not exist or might miraculously disappear if they refuse to acknowledge it.

For patients who have been dialyzed for some period of time and especially where there has been a history of good compliance in the past, noncompliance may signal moderate to severe depression which the patient finds difficult to express in a direct manner. Recurrent medical crises, the strain of the dialysis regimen, or family disturbances may cause the patient to question whether or not the prolongation of life is worth the effort. This ambivalence about "giving up" may first be seen as dietary indiscretion. In other cases, staff members may have misunderstood or ignored earlier signals for help and the patient is quite well aware that nothing is so likely to gain prompt attention, even if of a negative sort, as blatant noncompliance.

For patients who have already made the decision that life is not worthwhile, noncompliance can represent a passive or active suicide attempt. Those with strong moral or religious prohibitions against suicide may use dietary indiscretion to increase the risk of medical complications and death, while denying that they are playing an active role in precipitating such a crisis. Other patients may have in mind a concrete plan such as elevating potassium levels through diet and then refusing dialysis so that a fatal arrhythmia might be precipitated.

Staff Coping Devices

Just as patients may develop indirect and ineffective means of dealing with stress, professional staff, too, may develop techniques which help them to avoid direct confrontation with the stresses to which they are subjected. Perhaps one of the simplest and most common ways in which they do this is by *minimizing or ignoring physical and emotional distress*. At best, this tactic only temporarily alleviates staff discomfort, and it may have disastrous consequences for the patient whose serious medical problems are written off as hypochondriasis. Less assertive patients may withdraw if they feel they are not taken seriously, while others may escalate their complaints in a desperate attempt to gain attention, sympathy, or help.

At times, professionals may cope with dialysis unit stress by *interacting in an emotionally detached and mechanical manner* with patients who are seen not as people but as an assortment of medical problems: high BUN's, excessive weight gains, polycystic kidneys, etc. Such an approach can be extremely damaging to patients whose self-esteem has already been threatened by illness and who need support and reassurance that their worth as human beings is not diminished.

Labelling or pigeonholing is another technique used rather effectively by professionals. When confronted with some of the patient behaviors discussed in the preceding section, staff personnel make diagnoses rather than expending the time and energy necessary to determine reasons for the behavior. The patient is "passive-aggressive" or "manipulative" or "regressed." In addition to placing blame squarely on the patient while absolving the staff member from further responsibility, this tactic has an advantage in that the staff person may earn points for psychological sophistication.

Confronting and accusing patients is a time-honored way of dealing with the noncompliance that renal staff finds very troublesome and threatening, because it increases their workload and carries the implication that they have not properly educated their patients. "Your weight is up. You haven't been sticking to your diet," may help the staff person to feel self-righteous by placing blame on the patient, but it is not likely to help the patient solve whatever problem he has. In fact, this approach is most likely to lead to an argument of the form: "No I didn't"—"Yes you did"—"No I didn't," since the patient is almost forced into denying the indiscretion. A related tactic used by staff people is *lecturing*. Professionals like this approach because it makes them feel better by placing them in a position of benevolent power and authority and protects them from having to confront their own feelings of helplessness and fears that their treatment may have been inadequate in some way.

Given the significant discomfort that may be experienced by renal patients and staff and the human capacity, even propensity, for dealing indirectly and ineffectively with such discomfort, one may justifiably ask if there are any ways in which this dilemma can be resolved or alleviated. Experience on such units suggests that there probably are ways in which staff members can help themselves and their patients to cope more effectively, but there certainly appear to be no easy solutions. One approach, which sounds deceptively simple but in practice can be very difficult, is for staff members to view and respond to their colleagues and their patients as individual human beings with feelings, needs, expectations, and goals that are sometimes in conflict with their own. It is difficult to do this, however, unless the individuals involved are able to communicate their feelings and needs in a reasonably honest and straightforward manner. Investing some time and energy, therefore, in improving communication skills may yield significant benefits. In the section to follow, some aids to more effective communication will be discussed.

Facilitating Communication

Perhaps the first step we can take toward more effective communication is to *approach others with an open mind*. This means avoiding the pit-fall of instant diagnosis, admitting to ourselves and others that we don't have the answer to every question, and recognizing that we don't need to have all the answers. It also means acknowledging the fact that we are human beings and, therefore, fallible. Approaching colleagues or patients with the attitude that we have the only legitimate formulation of the problem or the only solution is likely to cut off communication before it has begun.

Further, we need to indicate to others our *receptiveness* to their point of view even if it is different from ours or not particularly pleasant to hear. This willingness is communicated not only by direct verbal expression but also by allowing others to state their views without interruptions or contradictions. Remaining receptive may be particularly difficult when we are hurried, when we are being criticized, or when patients communicate to us extreme emotional distress. For example, a common response to criticism is to defend ourselves rather than listening long enough to determine if there is some validity to the criticism or if the criticism might reflect anger or anxiety arising from sources unrelated to us. Common responses to patients who are very sad or who express suicidal thoughts include telling them to "cheer up" or that "things can't be all that bad." These responses, rather than reassuring patients or solving problems, tend to convey the message that we really don't want to hear what they are saying.

Receptiveness is communicated by body language as well as by words. We rarely fool others by saying we are willing to listen when our nervous mannerisms, wandering attention, and muscle tension betray the fact that we are in a hurry to get some place else or do something else. Patients are no exception and, indeed, may be quite sensitive to these nonverbal messages. Most of us have heard patients say, "I hate to bother the doctor with a lot of questions—he's so busy." If we cannot spend the time necessary with a patient, it is preferable to admit this openly and arrange to have the discussion at a later time when we are not so pressured.

A third aid to good communication is *patience*. Unfortunately, when time is limited and there is pressure to meet a schedule we may expect patients to conform to our schedule even in matters such as the discussion of sensitive personal material. Since it may be very difficult for the patient to raise such issues and they may be approached by a rather circuitous route, it is essential that he or she be given the time and extended attention necessary. Pushing patients to divulge such material or conveying our impatience by second-guessing them to move things along more quickly may be interpreted as a lack of interest and concern. There is, perhaps, no time when patience is of greater value than when dealing with the severely depressed patient. The withdrawal and slowed speech production commonly encountered in depression can prove extremely frustrating and yet, staying with the patient, even in silence, may be highly effective. In such situations, we must actively combat the societal taboo against silence and the feeling that unless we are talking we are not communicating. The ability to confront and control our own discomfort with silence can enhance our communication effectiveness.

Once we have conveyed our interest in and willingness to spend time with patients and they have begun to talk about matters that seriously concern them, we must be aware of the next step in the communication process: *active listening*. While simply being with patients and allowing them to vent their feelings may be helpful in certain situations, its usefulness is limited. And, if our mind is occupied by other concerns while we passively allow patients to ramble on, they are likely to sense the limitation of our involvement.

Active listening conveys to patients the fact that we are not only listening but are hearing what they say. This may be done in a number of ways. Much jest has been made of the psychiatrist's "Um-hum" response, but "Um-hums" interjected at appropriate points can help to let the patient know that we are attending and that our silence does not reflect preoccupation. Since assumptions that we understand what people are saying even when we may be far afield can disrupt communication, it is important that we check periodically to see if we are really following their train of thought. This may be done in part by restating in our own words what we think someone has said. It not only reassures the other person that we are making an active effort to understand them but also allows them to correct us if our perceptions have not been accurate. This technique, called *reflection*, has an added benefit in that the patient, hearing his thoughts expressed in a different way may get a clearer picture of the problem with which he or she is struggling. Reflection should not be confused with interpretation, which is telling the patient what we think is the "real" or hidden meaning of his thoughts. While interpretation can be a useful technique in the hands of the trained, skilled therapist, it is more likely to be abused than used effectively by individuals without appropriate training. Such interpretations may be far off target, conveying to patients that we do not understand them. In other instances, the perceptions may have some validity but touch on conflicts that patients are not willing to face at the time. In such cases, they may react with stout denial or anger and the flow of communication may be impeded because they feel that we are invading their privacy or trying to "read their minds."

An important issue affecting communication generally and especially that on the renal dialysis unit is *maintenance of confidentiality*. Where many professionals may treat a single patient, it is often important that information about patient problems confided to one staff member be passed on to other team members to insure appropriate treatment. However, if this is done without the patient's knowledge and consent, he or she may feel that the person who conveyed the information cannot be trusted with confidence. For this reason, it is very important that such problems be discussed with patients and the need for informing staff members be made clear. The patient may then be encouraged to speak directly with other staff or participate in a team meeting with the involved professionals so that the information can be shared. In some instances, the most practical route, and the one which the patient finds most comfortable, is for the staff member in whom the patient has confided to obtain his or her permission to share information with other staff members.

No matter how well our listening skills have been developed, patients are still likely to withdraw or become angry and dissatisfied if our intervention does not go beyond listening. Often, *taking appropriate action* is necessary. Allowing a patient to express anger about his lack of control over treatment procedures or decisions affecting his care will eventually be fruitless unless he is given an active role in treatment and decision making when this is possible. For the home dialysis patient who is upset because of family illness or marital discord related to the dialysis or other sources, understanding and verbal support may not be enough. Giving the patient and family a "vacation" by temporarily using center-based dialysis may free them to deal more rapidly and constructively with the crisis situation.

Similarly, it is not enough to understand that the patient's time is as valuable to him or her as the staff's time is to them and that expressions of anger about repeated delays in the dialysis schedule may be justified. Efforts must be made to identify sources of delay and correct them when possible so that patient expectations will not be constantly frustrated. Unavoidable delays and changes in schedule should be explained to patients with the recognition that their time is valuable and we may be inconveniencing them. While the time taken for such explanations may be seen by personnel as wasteful, in reality it is often efficient, taking far less time than that necessary to deal with an angry patient who feels his needs have been ignored.

An important way in which we can take action is by *providing appropriate information*. Questions from patients that seem to represent challenges to our authority, doubts about our competence, or overconcern with their medical status may reflect their need for information. In the medical setting, such information is in short supply at times. Perhaps even more frequently, it has been provided but in a form that is too technical, too detailed, too difficult, or too abbreviated for patients to understand. In some cases, information has been given in an appropriate manner, but because of emotional distress, the patient has not been able to understand. Therefore, questions should be given serious attention, even when they appear to be repetitious. Similarly, somatic complaints should be considered carefully, since they, too, may reflect a need for further information. Staff members sometimes think that they should ignore what they regard as unjustified physical complaints lest paying attention to them reinforce the complaints by conveying to the patient that the symptoms are serious. This tactic may actually lead to an exacerbation of the symptoms. By contrast, attending to the patient's complaints, evaluating them seriously, and providing information can prove to be reassuring and effective in reducing such complaints.

There are some guidelines to keep in mind when providing information to patients. First, it is important to make an estimate of their intelligence and sophistication so that information can be given at suitable levels. Noting the patient's level of education, speech patterns, and vocabulary and questioning them to find out what they currently understand can be most helpful in this respect. "Talking down" to a sophisticated patient can be as disruptive as "talking above the head" of the less sophisticated patient.

Once we have established a tentative level at which to convey information, it is important to check periodically to see if our initial impression was justified. Asking questions about the information we have given or asking patients to repeat in their own words what we have told them can serve as valuable "checks." Lest we overwhelm patients with more material than they can handle, it is probably wise to start with the most basic information and then encourage them to ask additional questions if they wish to know more details. Whenever possible, the use of basic English vocabulary is to be preferred to technical terms and professional jargon. The use of drawings, diagrams, and other audiovisual materials should not be overlooked as a means of conveying and clarifying information.

Another way in which we can facilitate communication is by *assisting patients with problem-solving.* This is probably one of the most fruitful approaches to the treatment of poor compliance. Excessive weight gains and poor blood chemistries may be approached as problems to be evaluated and remedied by patients and staff working together rather than alienating patients by accusing them of dietary indiscretion. This approach is not only more likely to yield solutions without causing patients to take a defensive stance, it also provides an opportunity to model an effective copying strategy. Asking patients for their opinions about the etiology of such problems may yield very valuable information. When they seem to be unaware of any reason for the problem, reviewing possible contributing factors may be helpful. In some cases, having patients keep medication or food diaries may serve to pinpoint the etiology of the problem. Once the source or sources of the problem have been identified, appropriate action may then be taken. This may involve education, reeducation, or investigating with the patient alternative ways of handling the situation.

Thus far, the discussion of communication has been primarily concerned with that between staff and patients. Not to be neglected is the important role of good intrastaff communications in reducing stress and enhancing treatment effectiveness on the unit. Maladaptive methods of dealing with stress affect patient treatment not only by influencing the way in which we interact with patients, but also the way in which we interact with each other. Often, when confronted with what appear to be insoluble problems in patient treatment, it is important for us to pause and examine our own contribution to the problems. Discussions of an informal nature with other staff members or formal, regularly scheduled interdisciplinary meetings can be helpful in this respect. Unfortunately, however, the primary focus of staff meetings is often patient problems.

Staff meetings can provide a forum for discussing frustrations arising from patient management, heavy workloads, and scheduling problems. They also provide an opportunity to share feelings of helplessness that often result from deterioration or death of patients. In addition, they can provide a safe and appropriate setting for airing conflicts related to staff responsibilities and functions, unit policies, and patient management and treatment planning.

When staff members can listen to each other and adopt a problem-solving approach to difficulties encountered in the work situation, stress may be significantly reduced in a number of ways. For example, open discussion of staff responsibilities with clarification of the roles to be played by members of the various professions on the unit can reduce stress arising from the "Double-Bind" phenomenon. Discussing and formulating consistent unit policies and individual treatment plans can reduce the anxiety and confusion that often result when guidelines are unclear. Patients, too, are likely to profit from consistency in treatment and feel more secure when the staff members work as a cohesive team. Furthermore, they will not be so tempted to play professionals against each other, thus reducing another source of stress.

At times, the unit staff will encounter problems which appear resistant to their best efforts to resolve them. In such cases, consultation with mental health professionals may prove helpful. Social workers, psychologists, and psychiatrists can offer not only expertise but new and different perspectives, since they are usually less intimately involved in the unit. In some cases, such as severely anxious, depressed, or suicidal patients, referrals to mental health professionals for direct intervention are necessary. Such patients may require not only special treatment skills but also expenditures of time that the unit staff can ill afford.

For those who are treated and those who work on the renal dialysis unit, there are no magic solutions to the abundant problems of the setting. Even modest reductions in conflict and stress require hard work, commitment, and patience. At times, maintaining the status quo appears to be the path of least resistance. Yet, problems ignored do not usually disappear; they grow and become more complex. Those who attempt to deal actively with them are likely to find that the time and energy invested have been well worthwhile.

REFERENCES

Alexander, L. The double-bind theory and hemodialysis. *Archives of General Psychiatry, 33,* 1353-1356, 1976.

Barofsky, I. Compliance, adherence and the therapeutic alliance: Steps in self-care. *Social Science and Medicine, 12,* 369-376, 1978.

Carpenter, J.O. Changing roles and disagreement in families with disabled husbands. *Archives of Physical Medicine and Rehabilitation, 55,* 272-274, 1974.

Czaczkes, J.W., and Kaplan-DeNour, A. *Chronic Hemodialysis as a Way of Life.* New York: Brunner/ Mazel, Inc., 1978.

Ford, C.V., and Castelnuovo, P. Hemodialysis and renal transplantation-psychopathological reactions and their management. In E.D. Wittkower and H. Warnes (Ed.), *Psychosomatic Medicine: Its Clinical Applications.* Hagerstown, Maryland: Harper & Row Pubs. Inc., 1977.

Moos, R.H., and Tsu, V.D. The crisis of physical illness: An overview. In R.H. Moos (Ed.), *Coping with Physical Illness.* New York: Plenum Medical Book Co., 1977.

Reichsman, F., and Levy, N.B. Problems in adaptation to maintenance hemodialysis. In N.B. Levy (Ed.), *Living or Dying: Adaptation to Hemodialysis.* Springfield, Illinois: Charles C Thomas, Publisher 1974.

Skipper, J., Fink, S., and Hallenbeck, P.N. Physical disability among married women: Problems in the husband-wife relationship. *Journal of Rehabilitation, 34,* 16-19, 1969.

Streltzer, J., Finkelstein, F., Feigenbaum, H., Kitsen, J., and Cohn, G.L. The spouse's role in home dialysis. *Archives of General Psychiatry, 33,* 55-58, 1976.

Chapter 11

COMMUNICATIONS IN A HEALTH CARE SETTING: THE STAFF PERSPECTIVE

LaFaye C. Sutkin

Clearly, communications of some sort occur all the time. When problems in communications are discussed, reference is usually intended to one of two major aspects of the communications process: what is communicated and the way in which it is communicated, or the quality of the communication. Because communication is an interpersonal interaction, there may always be at least two perspectives and interpretations involved. In the case of the health care setting, staff may have one view of the process, while patients have an entirely different perspective. In order for modification of maladaptive patterns of communication to occur, it is essential that each party in the communication process achieve the greatest possible understanding of the perspective of the other party. Appreciating the gains that might be expected from improved communications is also critical in providing the motivation for alteration of existing patterns of communication.

Most recently, increasing emphasis has been placed on the patients' rights to be informed of their condition, to understand the nature of the treatment or surgical procedures recommended for them, and to be participants in decisions regarding their medical management (Levin, 1978). The prevailing philosophy in health care psychology maintains that patients ultimately respond more favorably and learn to take greater personal responsibility for their rehabilitation in an environment that encourages their own motivation and initiative. Indeed, a growing body of research has accumulated which offers preliminary validation of that philosophy (Dodge, 1972; Dziurbejko & Larkin, 1978; Janis, 1958; Barofsky, 1978).

The Staff Perspective

There are health care workers, however, who feel such benefits do not necessarily accrue from adherence to "right to know" philosophies. Such feelings were expressed in a communications skill building workshop offered recently on the Spinal Cord Injury (SCI) Unit at the Cleveland Veterans Administration Medical Center. On this unit, administrative philosophies regarding patients' roles had evolved to one in which patients were provided with more information regarding their care and condition. It was, in part, to further enhance the communication process that the workshop was offered. During the first session, more senior staff members were asked to share their impression of the changes in communication patterns over the years. The expectation, of course, was that something of a testimonial would be tendered to the increased communication between staff and patients and the resulting informed participation of the patient in his rehabilitation program. Instead, one of the veteran nursing staff members unhesitatingly responded that communication was formerly better on the ward. When asked for some clarification of ways in which communication had formerly been "better," this nurse, and others as well, expressed the view that communication pathways had "broken down." The staff members offering this view were caring and dedicated nurses, so that the sincerity with which the opinions were given could not be questioned.

Veteran staff members recalled that communication once resulted in a desired response (usually compliance) rather than a debate. It was felt that patients had previously demonstrated greater respect for authority. When physicians ordered a surgical procedure, therapy, medication or schedule, the patients accepted those orders unquestioningly. The result was that patients seemed to work harder, i.e., participate in more therapies and activities, did not refuse to be turned (thereby reducing the number of decubiti incurred), and accepted ward routine in terms of awakening, bowel and bladder care, etc. It was clear from the discussion that the "communication pathway" referred to was the path from physician (or other professional) to the patient and that "better" referred to the consequences of the communication. The current situation on the unit was thought to permit debate, the result of which was, at times, noncompliance with the prescribed regimen. Furthermore, the consequences of noncompliance in this setting may be decubiti requiring months of debilitation, decreased strength, and reduced skill in self-care.

Prior patterns of communication were also viewed as "better" to the extent that one individual was prepared to take responsibility for a communication. In the past, "pathways" had a definite route from origin to destination with various members of the team representing stops along the way. It was very clear that orders originated with the physician and, regardless who delivered the message, questioning or objecting to anyone other than the physician was understood to be futile. Messages could be passed back to the physician, but no one of lesser authority was in a position to rescind an order or even provide answers for most questions.

In this respect, also, many staff members felt that the current philosophy resulted in "poorer" communications. The patient's right to more information was felt to place all members of the staff in a position of answering questions that these staff members felt (and were very likely taught) could be damaging to the patient. Further, they complained that responsibility had become more ambiguous. There was some consensus that, whereas in the past, nurses could not give information or accept refusals, exercising present options could result in criticism for assumption of too much responsibility or, failing to exercise those options might bring about criticism for refusing responsibility. It was the opinion of a number of individuals that they are "damned if they do and damned if they don't." In short, it was the view of the staff that this atmosphere of ambiguity represented less rather than more clarity in communications.

Finally, many conscientious nurses felt that communication was "better" when it was more pleasant or more palatable for the patient. Several long-time staff reported that, in the past, patients were not informed immediately that they would not walk again or that they might not function "normally" again sexually. These nurses expressed a conviction that such information was too discouraging to be discussed with the patient at the early stages of adjustment and might reduce the patient's motivation to work towards rehabilitation. Staff felt that the patient would learn these things in time, and, at such time, would be better prepared to cope.

Patients currently hospitalized were seen as more depressed and less motivated to pursue rehabilitation goals as a function of "dwelling on all that unpleasantness." In fact, one of the nurses related an incident in which a young man ceased eating regularly after having been told by a resident that he would not walk again. More frightening for those who recalled the case was the fact that the young man committed suicide while released for his next pass.

It is obviously easier to simply tell a patient that he or she must report for occupational therapy, or that it is time to be turned, or that he/she must eat or accept a surgical procedure. Explanations of what is to be done, how it will be carried out, why it is the wisest course, and what might be the possible side-effects and complications increase the work-load on a short-term basis. Moreover, the information related may, indeed, provoke an immediate increase in anxiety (Melamed & Siegel, 1975; Schmitt & Wooldridge, 1973) requiring the attention of the health care worker. Although considerable research has amassed to indicate that subsequent anxiety is reduced, that phase may be less apparent to the health care worker.

Resistance to informing the patient fully may derive from motivations other than ease or time-saving. Intensive questioning by patients or their families may be interpreted as a challenge to professional judgment for professionals who have devoted a large segment of their lives to learning special skills, either through lengthy formal education or extended on-the-job experience. The personal insult experienced by the professional is apparent in the comments that may be overheard after answering a barrage of questions, such as, "I don't know what he wants, we're doing all we can for him." It is clear, in such statements, that the professional has not considered the possibility that the patient simply wants to know more about what is happening to him.

Closely related to the feeling that questions imply challenges to professional judgment is the conviction that the patient does not possess sufficient knowledge or skill to make reasonable decisions regarding his or her care (Hulka, 1976). The professional who is particularly conscious of the extensive and intensive training required to be knowledgeable in his field may lose sight of the fact that his broad knowledge base is necessary in order to select the most salient data. It also requires considerable skill within an area to present facts in a nonevaluative way so that a patient is in a position to make reasonable decisions. All the skill and knowledge the professional acquires during training, however, cannot prepare him to make the decisions that involve the patient's personal values and attitudes. Patients may make reasonable decisions only when they can integrate all the relevant information into a framework of goals and attitudes (Wright, 1960).

Central to the issue over which nursing staff expressed concern is the fact that most dedicated health care workers feel stringent responsibility to "help" patients and "to make them better." It is important to remember that, for most persons working in a health care setting, a desire to help others was a primary consideration in the selection of vocational goals. The greatest difficulties arise, even for those subscribing wholeheartedly to the theory of "informed consent," when staff members must accept a patient's decision, knowing that the consequences of that decision will be detrimental or even fatal. Guided by the notion that success means improving the patient's condition in some way, the professional can only feel that he has failed if the patient refuses treatment.

Patient involvement may have been interpreted as detrimental in some cases because the health care worker measured progress as that which occurred within the area of his or her expertise. It is only natural that the field chosen by an individual is more likely to be the one that he regards as being of greatest significance to the rehabilitation program. For the most part, it is fortunate that this enthusiasm exists; it is a source of difficulty when the help offered is not wanted by the patient. In some cases, the patient may feel that he or she wishes to devote energy to some other aspect of rehabilitation, but, in other cases, patients may simply attach no importance to one dimension of rehabilitation.

Another conflict staff members may experience with regard to openness in communication arises over discussions of emotion-laden material. Concern that the patient cannot "handle" a fatal diagnosis or the knowledge that he will never walk again or be able to produce children is a source of apprehension for many health care workers. Moreover, even if the patient is informed, staff may feel that "dwelling" on such unpleasantness is detrimental (Hinton, 1971; Sanders & Kardinal, 1977).

This concern over emotion-laden material may reflect concern for the patient. In some instances, however, reluctance to communicate unpleasant information to the patient may reflect the health care worker's personal discomfort with the subject matter (Epstein, 1975; Uustal, 1978). It is possible that the topic relates to the worker's own fears. It may be that the particular case too strongly resembles one in which the worker was personally involved. Or the worker may feel too similar to the patient, so that he is forced to confront his own vulnerability. When the staff member is aware of these obstacles to communication, it is usually no problem to pass the task along to a coworker until these feelings have been worked out. Often, unfortunately, the feelings are not entirely apparent to the individual experiencing them, so that incomplete or distorted communications result.

Fear of "getting too close" to patients may be among the feelings that stand as a block to openness (Morgan, Hohmann, & Davis, 1974; Conroe, 1974). For those individuals in the health care field who can only cope with catastrophic disease and injury by depersonalizing the patient, the requirement to provide open and complete information may be highly threatening.

Finally, tension and conflict among staff may introduce obstacles to openness with patients. Where staff is not certain of the limits of their authority to speak to patients or when staff disagree over the diagnosis or treatment of the patient, the patient may be caught in the middle. Health care professionals have traditionally subscribed to the notion that contradictory opinions rendered to the patient introduce unnecessary anxiety and undermine confidence.

In summary, it is not always easy to comply with the fiat to provide complete and accurate information to the patient. There are genuine complications that may arise as a result of communicating openly with a patient and as a result of considering the patient's opinions. Further, there are traditional and long-standing beliefs concerning communication patterns that must be countered with convincing evidence to the contrary before they will be dispelled.

In general, discussion has focused on what is communicated, or the content of the communications. However, the quality of communications may be equally important. Communications in health care facilities are generally imagined to be full of warmth, support, gratitude, and respect. It is usually a surprise to patients, staff, and visitors to find that communications can deteriorate to the point that they are best characterized as hostile, abusive, resentful, patronizing, or guilt-inducing. Even when such overt communication characteristics are not present, positive communications may be absent because patients or staff have withdrawn from each other. In order to understand some of the factors underlying the deterioration in communication patterns that occasionally occurs between staff and patients, it is important to recognize that each party brings certain attitudes, expectations, personality, and coping styles into every interaction (Uustal, 1978; Means & Akridge, 1978).

It is often the case that unrealistic expectations and irrational beliefs block direct and satisfying communications between individuals. In health care settings, staff may also bring with them certain attitudes and beliefs that may never be directly expressed but which may operate to distort all communications (Ellis, 1975; Means & Akridge, 1978).

The opportunity, indeed the responsibility, to help others, particularly the ill, is probably the major expectation of individuals who select health care careers. But helping is a two-way process requiring another individual who is prepared to accept that help. Both the patients who will not accept help and the patients who cannot accept help may be seen as frustrating the health care worker's efforts and interfering with the fulfillment of that worker's expectations. The patient who will not accept the help may be perceived as rejecting the helper, thereby evoking hostility. Similarly, the patient who is beyond help, i.e. terminally ill, etc., may evoke hostility to the dismay of the staff person experiencing those feelings, because his condition has deprived the health care worker of the opportunity to help (Kübler-Ross, 1970).

A similar expectation, that patients who are seriously ill or injured deserve to be cared for and waited upon, may also create obstacles to straightforward and direct communications. For example, a particularly difficult issue for nursing assistants arises when rehabilitation patients object to assuming greater responsibility for self-care, accusing their caretakers of shirking the jobs they are paid to perform. It is natural that such accusations might provoke hostility in the recipient, but guilt and personal discomfort may also ensue. Nursing assistants who react sympathetically to a patient may believe that the patient is entitled to be served. Furthermore, conscientious but overworked aides may recognize the truth in the patient's claim that his self-care will reduce the work load. For some aides, the fact that increasing responsibility is good for the patient may be overshadowed by feelings of guilt. In such a case, the aide is likely to attempt to defend himself against the attack and the patient may succeed in diverting the conversation from the real issue, i.e. his rehabilitation.

Frequently, health care staff expect that the person who is helped will appreciate that help and express gratitude to the helper. A common complaint registered by staff was that patients on the spinal cord injury unit seemed entirely lacking in gratitude for care provided. It was observed that patients who received the most intensive care were most likely to complain of inattention. There are, of course, numerous reasons that patients may not be able to feel gratitude. Even if gratitude is felt, patients may feel that expression of gratitude will add to their vulnerability. In many cases, communications may break down between a staff member and a patient because the patient has failed to fulfill a contract which specifies gratitude in return for care—a contract of which the patient is unaware.

All levels of employees in health care facilities have traditionally been accorded some respect and prestige by the community for their service. It is, therefore, reasonable to expect that a number of individuals enter the health care field in order to gain some of that respect and status. Anger, disagreement, even certain forms of humor displayed by patients may be seen as proof of lack of respect and have produced resentment among some employees. One employee justified her anger at a patient on the basis of his use of her first name. She admitted that she had not confronted the patient with the fact that she preferred to be addressed more formally; she had assumed that the act of calling a health care worker by a first name had a universal meaning, i.e. that respect was not felt for that worker. The possibility of pleasant interactions between the two individuals did not exist as long as assumptions were acted upon and not communicated.

A major basis for the respect given health care workers is the fact that their work carries with it considerable responsibility. The jobs of health care workers quite literally involve life and death matters. Persons willing to assume such responsibility frequently possess leadership qualities that incline them to take charge of a situation and remain in control (Yura, 1973). A group of patients considered difficult by responsible staff were those who ignored decisions reached by authorities regarding scheduling and routine. According to staff, there are always a few individuals who demand that modifications in routine be made, even though the changes sought appear too trivial to be of any consequence. Staff tends to interpret these demands as challenges to authority and as attempts to disrupt the smooth functioning of the unit.

While some staff believe that their decisions should be unquestioned, others hold the belief that the patient is always right and that the staff has no rights. This belief (irrational, when carried to the extreme) leads some health care workers to ignore offensive or abusive remarks, inappropriate behavior, sexual overtures, etc. Acting upon this belief, staff may communicate to patients, unwittingly, that the patient is no longer important enough to cause offense or that he no longer must set limits on his behavior (Morgan, Hohmann, & Davis, 1974).

Patients are entitled to be sad or frightened, but not angry or demanding. Several nurses commented on the hostility they experience after a day of continuously answering the calls of a patient. Comments were made such as, "I don't know why he asks for all those things, he just likes to see us run," or "He waits until we've left the room to remember that there is something else he wants," and "He never asks for two things at once." With other patients, staff members may engage in frequent verbal battles over issues known to be trivial. These situations persist because staff has difficulty recognizing that emotional responses to injury may be communicated through demanding or angry behavior (Epstein, 1975; Hanson, 1974).

Many health care workers have preconceived attitudes that patients are childlike. The origins of these attitudes are easily understood when the frequency with which one hears the expression, "Men are just like children when they're sick" is considered. The effects of the notion that patients are like children, however, may be patronizing communications through which the patient comes to believe that he no longer has adult status. Consequently, some patients may fulfill expectations and behave in child-like ways.

Finally, health care is an action-oriented discipline and, often, its providers expect that when there is a problem, there should be a solution. Health care workers frequently feel that being apprised of a patient's problems means that they must *do something* about that problem. In the case of patients who communicate that they are depressed or anxious, staff members often feel compelled to "cure" the depression. During the workshops, many staff members sought guidance in coping with patients who were obviously very depressed or frightened. Individual staff related a variety of reactions and responses they typically gave to depressed patients. Some reported attempts to talk the patient out of his negative feelings; others acknowledged that they withdrew from patients who too openly displayed such feelings in order to avoid a sense of inadequacy; and one staff member admitted "babying" patients who are "down." The impulse to "make it better," in the case of negative feelings, may clearly interfere with staff's capacity to listen to the patient. Thus, various expectations and assumptions of health care workers may serve as an obstacle, not only in their capacity to communicate warmth and support to the patient, but also in their capacity to listen to the patient.

Understanding the development of maladaptive communications in the health care setting also requires an understanding of the patient's psychological stresses and the way that these may interact with staff needs and expectation to produce snarls in the communication process. In fact, attempting to better understand the patient is the first stop in the communication process. Patients hospitalized for almost any reason are likely to be frightened and anxious. They are also likely to be depressed, at least mildly. They have had their lives disrupted in most cases, and their presence in a hospital is tantamount to an admission that they are helpless to cope with their condition alone. In addition to depression, this helplessness and dependence upon others often produces in patients a sense that they have lost control over their lives. During hospitalization, most patients undergo a role change: For the husband and father, the role of provider and caretaker is reversed; for the nurturant mother, the role of nurtured patient must be temporarily endured, etc. Individuals experiencing all of these changes as well as the effects of physical crisis are inclined to be more self-absorbed than would usually be the case, and may, therefore, be less sensitive to the needs of others. Added to this self-absorption is the fact that persons who feel ill or are in pain are inclined to have a lower threshold for irritability. For most hospitalized patients, these stresses are present in mild form, but hospitalization usually brings about fairly rapid recovery, so that life may return to normal in a short time (Mayer & Peterson, 1978; Eisenberg, 1978).

On the other hand, for spinal cord injured patients whose hospitalization is longer-term and whose condition is more debilitating, these stresses are more potent and, to these, others may be added. As is true of other conditions, such as ulcers or heart disease, spinal cord injury has been associated with the presence of a number of demographic characteristics that affect the patient's handling of stress. Although these characteristics do not hold true in all cases of spinal cord injury, they do appear frequently enough to influence the character of a spinal cord injury ward. These patients are likely to be young, vigorous, and active. Undoubtedly, such individuals more often engage in activities that lead to serious injury. Males acquire spinal cord injuries more often than do females and these males are more likely to be daring, risk-taking, and generally "macho" than would be expected in the population. Since more thoughtful and reflective individuals are better able to anticipate and avert serious injuries, spinal cord injured patients tend more often to be impulsive and fail to see their role in producing negative outcomes. Similarly, in communications, such individuals are unlikely to understand that their behavior can be responsible for negative behaviors of staff.

Compounding the effects of demographic characteristics of SCI patients and the stresses of hospitalization in general are the unique stresses placed on the patient as a direct result of spinal cord injury. There is a dramatic sense of loss that accompanies paralysis of limbs, a sense of loss comparable to that experienced by persons who have lost loved ones or who have had a limb amputated. Further, this loss is typically incurred suddenly, preventing any prolonged anticipation and adjustment. Typically, patients experience some cycle of adaptation that includes such states as anxiety, denial, anger, and depression (Eisenberg, 1977; Sanders & Kardinal, 1977). Unless these emotional states become extreme or excessive in duration, they may be considered appropriate and adaptive. Health care workers responding to a need to "do something" to reverse these states may communicate to a patient, however, that his emotional reaction is inappropriate. In addition, staff may perceive a failure to get better as a professional failure or as rejection by the patient.

Spinal cord injured patients have usually experienced dramatic alterations in their social roles, and for these patients, the change is essentially permanent in that they will be unable to return to some activities that defined their prior roles. In addition to the change in roles that results from loss of mobility and sexual function, roles that had been previously defined by an individual's body image must be redefined to include physical changes and a wheelchair. In the process of redefining a role for himself, the patient may behave in ways that seem to staff to be manipulative, aggressive, or offensive. For example, a patient may examine the effectiveness of assuming the role of "a cripple" to determine how effectively that role will meet his needs. Whether a staff member sees this behavior as demanding or feels that the patient is appropriate in this role will determine the manner in which the staff member communicates with the patient. And, the way in which the staff member communicates will greatly affect the patient's decisions regarding his role (Eisenberg, 1977).

Although hospitalization always requires that patients cede some control over their lives, spinal cord injured patients must cope with an enormous loss of control. In the absence of basic control over bowel and bladder function as well as lack of control over getting up or staying in bed, tremendous dependency on staff is a necessity, particularly in early stages of injury. Dependency is likely to be extremely distressing for patients whose personality style before injury was somewhat "macho" and controlling. Patients may attempt a variety of maneuvers, such as rearranging schedules or requesting special privileges, in order to assess how much control they may still exert over their environment. Excessive demands may be the technique through which patients learn whether others are prepared to meet their needs and through which patients learn the limits of their control. Anger, demands, and passivity-dependency may all be ways of testing limits.

If the patient has sustained an injury as a result of engaging in a dangerous activity or as a consequence of impulsive and careless actions, guilt feelings may exist. Other patients, whose injuries have entirely accidental origins, occasionally interpret the injury as punishment for some earlier "sin." On the other hand, many patients are likely to see others as agents of their misfortune. Anger at fate, God or anyone who might be held responsible is common. In order to cope with these feelings, anger may be directed at whoever is available as a target. Such expressions of anger serve as a pressure valve for the patient. For the staff member who becomes the victim of this anger, the nonspecific nature of the anger is not apparent. If the staff member expected gratitude and respect for his attention to the patient, the role of scapegoat to the patient's frustration is likely to produce hurt, frustration, and resentment.

Many patients, but particularly "macho" males, find it difficult or embarrassing to express softer emotions, such as fear or sadness. Patients may vent their depression indirectly, through anger or unreasonable demands. In some cases, patients may be genuinely unconscious that their behavior communicates anger or that they are being excessively demanding. When staff respond to the patient's anger with hostility or resentment, the patient is likely to feel more helpless, dependent, and depressed and, as a result, increase the angry behavior. Patients who find their efforts to organize their world around themselves frustrated after a major disruption are more likely to make new demands or to be more forceful in making the same requests if they perceive that their initial efforts are unproductive. Some patients will persist in escalating demands until they feel that they have hit upon an effective approach. Therefore, it is possible that a staff member who ignores the requests of patients in order to communicate to a patient that he should reduce his demands may have the reverse effect.

It is not at all surprising to find that patients who have suffered a tragedy of the dimensions of a spinal cord injury are temporarily self-centered and unable to spare any concern for others while adjusting to their injury. In many cases, patients see themselves singled out for misfortune and expect to be compensated for their losses by the rest of the world. Staff expecting patients to satisfy some of their emotional needs, such as expressing gratitude and offering respect, may be trying to drink from a particularly dry well.

In the face of these several obstacles to openness between patients and staff, what advantages may be expected to accrue from greater openness with patients? One of the obvious advantages from disclosure is the resulting improvement in interpersonal climate. Many interpersonal difficulties may be circumvented by providing patients with complete information. Suspicion and distrust of staff by patients is likely to be reduced when "all the cards are on the table." Moreover, patients are less likely to see staff as adversaries than they might when information is withheld. Apart from the fact that an improved interpersonal climate is simply more pleasant, there is some data which supports tangible benefits to patients' rehabilitation deriving from better interpersonal climates (Moos, 1975).

Although emotional reactions such as depression, anxiety, and hostility are to be expected in response to catastrophic injuries or illness, investigators have found that providing sufficient information and open discussion of important topics may significantly affect the intensity of those states (Levy, 1973; Dziurbejko & Larkin, 1978; Lindemann, 1972). Understanding as much as is possible about one's condition permits the individual to begin to adjust and accept things as they will be. Uncertainty delays those adjustments and promotes higher levels of anxiety (Light & Kleiber, 1978; Wright, 1960).

A free flow of information between staff and patients may also carve away many of the blocks to compliance in the health care setting (Barofsky, 1978). In an atmosphere that is perceived as authoritarian, the patient may lose sight of the fact that the program was designed to benefit him or her, and rebellion against authority may lead the patient to subvert his own recovery. Furthermore, patients often supply their own answers in the absence of adequate information. The result may be an interpretation of available data that is more serious than is actually the case. Any effort may be regarded as futile by a patient who regards his case as hopeless, but this sense of hopelessness may not be communicated to a staff that is not regarded as honest, so that misconceptions may not be corrected. Conversely, patients who are fully informed of their condition, their alternatives, and the consequences are in a position to make reasonable decisions *and* are unlikely to find a reason to rebel. Staff members who have noticed that patients refuse treatment after learning that they have the right to do so may be observing a test by the patient of those rights. In such cases, the patients are likely to slowly assume responsibility only when they have satisfied themselves that they are in control. Several groups participating in the communication workshop reported an incident in which a patient refused turns for two or three days immediately after having been informed of his rights. Each group, when questioned, recalled that the patient subsequently requested that his turns be resumed on schedule. In this case, there were no decubiti incurred and the patient learned that he was in control.

While it is true that patients may invoke their privilege to refuse treatment even when objectively maladaptive consequences follow, health care workers must bear in mind that those privileges are granted once the patient is discharged from the hospital. A patient who persistently refuses turns in the hospital is unlikely to submit to turns at home. Indeed, if turns have been a major issue during hospitalization, the freedom from control perceived at discharge is likely to be seen as an opportunity to rebel. In most cases, patients will not pursue options to a point that is hazardous, but, when this occurs, it is probably preferable that it occur in the hospital where remedial steps may be taken promptly. In any case, the more stringently patients have been controlled by staff, the greater is the likelihood that they will test that authority when they go home. Ultimately, if a rehabilitation program has been effective, the patient will assume increasing responsibility for his care while still in the hospital, and discharge will serve only as a point in the passage of responsibility from staff to patient. Although noncompliance may be the result of many factors, it is unlikely that compelling patients to comply will eliminate any of those factors. In fact, studies such as that conducted by Hulka (1976) suggest that overall compliance in a health care setting increases when patients are given a clearer understanding of all the facts.

It is certainly true that some patients, given options, will not elect to pursue active and demanding rehabilitation programs voluntarily. Health care teams, however, must consider established priorities. Is it more important for the patient to have attained an understanding that a number of options exist and that the choices are his? Health care teams must also consider what they wish to communicate to patients: Do we wish to communicate that rehabilitation is something that is done to him or her, or do we wish the patient to know that rehabilitation offers an opportunity for the patient to do something for himself? Rehabilitation in the latter case becomes something that the patient has achieved and may continue to achieve. While overwhelming gratitude from a successful rehabilitation patient is gratifying, how much more gratifying is the patient who begins his almost new life with the self-confidence that derives from successful accomplishments of self-selected goals (Wright, 1960).

Finally, it is an obvious benefit to the patient and staff that the patient understand as much as possible by the time of discharge, since the patient must, at that time, assume responsibility for his care and the monitoring of his own condition. Despite the arguments that patients lack the knowledge and skill to understand their condition and what is being done to them, it is often the case that the same patient will be ushered into a room just prior to discharge and given a "crash course" in precisely the same material he was denied access to earlier. This information would seem to be more relevant to the patient as he is experiencing the initial impact during hospitalization. Moreover, the opportunity for misunderstandings to be elicited and dispelled is far greater if the patient has the opportunity to test his understanding under trained supervision. Finally, the repetition of procedures over months of rehabilitation is more likely to produce permanent learning than is a sketchy summary provided at the end of hospitalization (Romankiewicz, Gotz, Capelli, & Carlin, 1978; Hulka, 1976).

Even if the patient has been fully informed and has been allowed to set his goals and make input into his rehabilitation program, the quality of communications have the capacity to hamper his emotional rehabilitation and personal growth. Conversely, a rehabilitation setting in which interpersonal communications convey understanding, warmth, support, and mutual respect has the potential of facilitating a psychological adjustment that is more positive and adaptive than was the case prior to injury (Mayer & Peterson, 1978).

Clearly, a more pleasant atmosphere is relaxed and permits energy to be devoted to rehabilitation that might be diverted into conflict. Staff sometimes forgets that only one-third of their day is spent in the hospital; whereas, the long-term patient is confined to the setting round the clock. Continuous antagonism drains energy (Conroe, 1974).

In addition, positive communications may reduce the intensity and duration of depression. If interactions are negative or frustrating, patients may be left with a greater sense of helplessness. The psychological sense of powerlessness added to physical loss of power may prolong or deepen normally occurring depressive or anxious states (Wright, 1960).

Probably the most significant benefit the patient may derive from staff's positive communications is a positive self-image. Patients who have acquired a spinal cord injury have massive changes to assimilate. SCI patients frequently have scars which alter their physical appearance, and inevitably lose muscle mass in paralyzed muscle groups. The result may be as extreme as a "Charles Atlas" turning into a "ninety-pound weakling." Not only do patients look different to themselves, the world, seen at the height of a wheelchair, looks different to them. The very activities that may have previously defined the patient for himself, for example, his identity as a steel worker, "bike" rider, athlete, dancer, lover, or head of household, have been undermined. The patient is faced with the task of reestablishing an identity for the helpless body that confronts him when he looks in the mirror. The manner in which a new self-image is built is very similar to the way children evolve a self-image, that is, from information they receive from those around them. The persons most consistently present to provide SCI patients with feedback as to the way they are seen and reacted to are staff (Ostwald, 1977). In the optimal situation, feedback from staff will provide the patient with a reflection of himself as a competent, fully functional adult who is able to control his own life, but he must be subject to the same social rules and limits as those around him (Wright, 1960; Hanson, 1974).

Since it is the goal of staff to realize optimal rehabilitation, both physically and emotionally, staff is rewarded for efforts at improving the quality of communications when this occurs. More direct benefits may also be seen by staff. Among the consequences that might be expected from enhanced communications are the following: better compliance by patients, reduced demands from patients who feel in control of important aspects of their lives, fewer angry outbursts from adult patients who know the importance of respect first-hand (Christensen, 1978; Wright, 1960).

Understanding the many benefits that might be expected to derive from improved communications in a health care setting does not, however, remove the obstacles to the realization of ideal communications. Each patient and each setting is unique and requires individualized efforts to enhance communications, but there are some measures and techniques that seem applicable to most settings. It may be that the first obligation health care staff have in facilitating optimal communications is to clarify the goals of the patient and staff (Morgan, Hohmann, & Davis, 1974). It is unfortunate when staff and patients are committed to working towards separate and distinct goals; it is not necessarily a rare occurrence. Furthermore, problems are compounded when both staff and patients assume that their goals are identical and, yet, find themselves conflicting at every stage of the program. An explicit discussion of goals (as soon as the patient has been given sufficient information to formulate goals) is a major step in cutting through subsequent blocks to open communication. In those cases in which the patient elects goals that are contradictory to the rehabilitation process or to some phase of that process, staff members may feel disappointment, but they may be spared much of the frustration produced by pushing a patient who will not move. In addition, some of the innocent deceptions that are occasionally practiced to "seduce" the patient may be averted. It may be true that a patient *compelled* to follow a program might more completely meet staff goals; is it staff goals that count? The law has stated for us that it is the patient's goal that must be pursued. This remains true even in the case of the ultimate disparity of goals: The patient may exercise his option to choose death as a goal, while the staff maintains a commitment to fulfill their responsibility to preserve life (Wright, 1960).

The second major step in improving communications requires that staff convey all available information to patients honestly and simply. Determining the detail with which information is given obviously depends upon accurate assessment of the patient's capacity to understand and his desire to listen. Patients generally monitor what they are ready to hear and provide feedback to the professional as to the appropriateness of the information. Receiving feedback, however, demands that the professional attend to questions and reactions of the patient (Epstein, 1975). The task of reducing technical information to a level that may be understandable to a layman can be very difficult but is not impossible. Illustrations may often cut through the barriers erected by language, but even with illustrations it is important to check out with the patient the extent to which he has understood the information he has been given. Frequently, patients will indicate understanding when, in fact, their understanding is so poor they cannot begin to ask the appropriate questions. Patients who are asked to describe in their own words what they understand concerning their condition or a procedure often reveal substantial gaps and frightening distortions.

Communications between staff and patients depend significantly on a third factor, that is, communications among staff members. It would be contrary to the philosophy of open communications to withhold information from a patient because a view is not consistently held by all of staff. An equally ungenuine approach would have staff members deciding on a unified statement for purposes of informing the patient, while continuing to privately disagree. It is preferable that staff be in communication with each other, so that they are aware that conflicting views exist. In this case, alternative possibilities may be presented to the patient. The fact that medicine is not an exact science is much more widely accepted today than in the past, and patients are generally capable of understanding that differences of opinion occur. A patient who knows that both theories are being explored may feel secure in the knowledge that his staff will consider multiple possibilities before arriving at a definitive picture. On the other hand, a patient who is given opposing points of view by staff in ways that deny alternate possibilities is likely to be skeptical about his treatment and is more likely to experience anxiety.

Finally, staff must consider the patient's opinions when making any decision. If patient's opinions are not included in the decision-making process, much of the communication process is meaningless. For example, if a patient has been asked to share his goals with staff and has been informed of every detail of the diagnostic workups and treatment process but is ignored when he decides that a brace will not fit his vocational life-style as well as a wheelchair, he is likely to feel more deceived than if he had been excluded altogether (Wright, 1960).

Providing complete, accurate and clear information to the patient and including the patients opinions in decision-making are essential ingredients in improving the quality of communication as well. Open communications and informed consent are necessary to give credibility to the respect and support and acceptance that characterize rewarding patient-staff interactions. As mentioned previously, positive communications do not occur without effort, even in an environment that is open; effort is necessary to overcome some of the obstacles in the way of mutually satisfying communications. The first, and probably most important, step that staff can take to enhance communications is to listen to patients. Listening is a skill, and, like other skills, must be learned and refined. In order to listen, it is necessary to spend some time with the patient. There are many health care workers who regret that the demands on their time prevent any extended contact. However, it is sometimes the case that a few minutes spent listening to each patient can reduce enough of the demands for unnecessary attention to allow for listening time.

Having allowed for listening, there are often individuals (in and out of hospital settings) who find it difficult to tolerate silence. Frequently, patients are "talked to" rather than "talked with" by health professionals and, when the patient is offered an opportunity to ask a question, he is often given only moments to reply. If a patient has something important or personal to say, it is quite likely to take him a minute or two to formulate his communication. Becoming comfortable with silence is, therefore, another step in learning to listen to the patient. And a silence that indicates a willingness to hear from the patient can communicate understanding and respect for the patient.

However, there is more to listening than simply hearing the words that are spoken. Too often patients, particularly male patients, are uncomfortable discussing feelings of depression, sadness, loss, fear, etc. It is often necessary to listen empathically. That is, to listen in a way that puts the listener in the shoes of the speaker. Empathy enables the listener to imagine what he might feel in the same situation. The listener who understands how he would feel is usually in a position to hear the feelings hidden in the words of the speaker. If those feelings do not seem to be expressed, the listener can suggest how he would feel and wonder if the patient might not be experiencing similar feelings. It is imperative to remember, however, that the same situation may have different meanings for different individuals. For that reason, we cannot know except as the patient chooses to tell us, exactly what his feelings are. Nonetheless, inquiring about feelings in this way may free the patient to correct staff and give voice to the feelings he is experiencing (Uustal, 1978).

It is quite possible that health care workers fail to listen for or hear feelings expressed because they feel that, if those feelings are heard, they are obligated to do something, to correct the situation. In the case of depression following an accident that resulted in quadriplegia, the health care worker may accurately perceive that he cannot correct the depression, that he cannot make the person happy (at least not immediately). It is perhaps because complaints of bad feelings are viewed as comparable to complaints about a broken leg that people so often respond by telling the person that they "shouldn't feel that way," that they "have so much to live for," that they "will get better," or that "they shouldn't dwell on all that unhappiness." Listening to feelings requires acceptance of those feelings. Very often, patients experience tremendous relief as a result of describing their feeling, believing that the other person understands those feelings, and observing that the other person does not consider the patient weak or spineless for his inability to "keep a stiff upper lip." The feelings that are denied a right to existence by others do not go away, they are, in fact, more likely to increase, since outlets for ventilating them appear blocked.

As difficult as it may be to hear the sadness reflected in a story of former daring antics from a macho young man, it is even more difficult to hear the feelings of anxiety and fear which may be expressed as anger directed at the listener. Similarly, it is difficult to be sensitive to the need for company and reassurance when it is expressed in the forms of frequent complaints and demands. However, for many individuals, the expression of anger is far more acceptable than the expression of such "unmanly" feelings as anxiety or fear.

In addition to feelings, patients may communicate their wishes or their questions indirectly, requiring empathic listening to interpret. Some patients may consider it inappropriate to complain about their care but express their dissatisfaction in other ways. It is sometimes necessary to look for a communication of dissatisfaction in a series of maladaptive behaviors. On the other hand, there are other ways to approach many of these particular difficulties in communications. Patients may be indirect in their approaches to staff because they perceive staff as being indirect or dishonest in their communications with patients. An atmosphere in which the staff speaks with patients in straightforward and genuine ways is likely to produce patients who will also be direct.

Indirect communications may often result from one or more irrational beliefs or unrealistic expectations. For example, when staff expectations are not met by a patient (who may be oblivious to the expectation), the staff member may feel that the patient has indirectly communicated a lack of respect or appreciation. In response to the perceived slight, the staff member may indirectly communicate to the patient that he is of little importance by consistently caring for other patients first. Unwarranted assumptions and irrational beliefs may also lead to more overtly negative communications. An important technique staff members can apply to communication problems that may have developed with a patient is an examination of the process leading to poor communications. Only when staff is aware of the beliefs, assumptions, and expectations on which they operate can they begin to untangle some of the snarled communication patterns. Awareness of an underlying assumption enables the staff member to check-out with the patient the accuracy of the interpretation of a behavior (Means & Akridge, 1978).

Providing feedback to patients requires a willingness to be genuine without being judgmental. Patients, like staff, benefit from expressions of appreciation, praise or respect. When these feelings are expressed by staff in circumstances that are appropriate, the positive behaviors tend to be reinforced. A side-benefit which may (but cannot be expected to) accrue from offering positive statements to patients is that patients are more likely to return compliments and appreciation.

On the other hand, genuine statements regarding the *concrete* behavior that negatively affects staff can, if communicated in a *nonblameful way*, inform the patient of the way he is perceived and of the limits of appropriate behavior. Blameful criticism tends to have several effects: it arouses hostility, causes individuals to become defensive, and gives the person a sense of worthlessness. Rarely does such criticism change the behavior.

Communications characterized by openness and honesty are more likely to increase the patient's willingness to communicate with staff. In general, communicating with patients is like communicating with anyone: If what is communicated is direct, honest, and genuine, if a willingness to listen and a desire to understand is demonstrated, and if a readiness to accept and respect the other individual exists, communications will be optimal.

REFERENCES

Barofsky, I. Compliance, adherence and the therapeutic alliance: Steps in the development of self-care. *Social Science and Medicine, 12,* 369-376, 1978.

Christensen, D. B. Drug-taking compliance: A review and synthesis. *Hospital Services Research, 13,* 171-181, 1978.

Conroe, R. M. The psycho-ecological approach: A new model for psychologists functioning on Spinal Cord Injury Service. *Rehabilitation Psychology, 21,* 34-38, 1974.

Dodge, J. S. What patients should be told: Patients and nurses beliefs. *American Journal of Nursing, 72,* 1852-1854, 1972.

Dziurbejko, M., and Larkin, J. C. Including the family in pre-operative teaching. *American Journal of Nursing, 78,* 1892-1895, 1978.

Eisenberg, M. G. *Psychological Aspects of Physical Disability: A Guide for the Health Care Educator.* New York: National League for Nursing, 1977.

Ellis, A., and Harper, R. A. *A New Guide to Rational Living.* Englewood Cliffs, New Jersey: Prentice-Hall, Inc., 1975.

Epstein, C. *Nursing the Dying Patient.* Reston, Virginia: Reston Publishing Co., Inc., 1975.

Hanson, R. W. The psycho-ecological approach to Spinal Cord Injury rehabilitation: A behaviorist perspective. *Rehabilitation Psychology, 21,* 39-43, 1974.

Hinton, J. Assessing the views of the dying. *Social Science and Medicine, 5,* 37-43, 1971.

Hulka, B. S. Communication, compliance, and concordance between physician and patient with prescribed medication. *American Journal of Public Health, 66,* 847-853, 1976.

Janis, I. L. *Psychological Stress: Psychoanalytic and Behavioral Studies of Surgical Patients.* New York: John Wiley & Sons, Inc., 1958.

Kübler-Ross, E. The care of the dying: whose job is it? *Psychiatry in Medicine, 1,* 103-107, 1970.

Levin, L. Self-care: An emerging component of the health care system. *Hospital and Health Services Administration, 23,* 17-26, 1978.

Levy, N. B. Fatal illness: Should the patient be told? *Medical Insight, 3,* 20-23, 1973.

Light, L., and Kleiber, N. Interactive research in a health care setting. *Social Science and Medicine, 12,* 193-198, 1978.

Lindemann, C. A. Nursing intervention with the pre-surgical patient: The effects of structured and unstructured pre-operative teaching. *Nursing Research, 21,* 12-19, 1972.

Mayer, G., and Peterson, C. W. Theoretical framework for coronary care nursing education. *American Journal of Nursing, 78,* 1208-1211, 1978.

Means, R., and Akridge, R. L. Psychological and behavioral adjustment: A model of healthy personing. *Journal of Rehabilitation, 44,* 24-30, 1978.

Melamed, B. G., and Siegel, L. J. Reduction of anxiety in children facing hospitalization and surgery by use of filmed modeling. *Journal of Consulting and Clinical Psychology, 43,* 511-521, 1975.

Moos, R. H. Assessment and impact of social climate. In P. McReynolds (Ed.), *Advances in Psychological Assessment.* San Francisco: Jossey-Bass Publishers, 1975.

Morgan, E. D., Hohmann, G. W., and Davies, J. E. Psychosocial rehabilitation in VA spinal cord injury centers. *Rehabilitation Psychology, 21,* 3-27, 1974.

Ostwald, P. F. *Communication and Social Interaction: Clinical and Therapeutic Aspects of Human Behavior.* New York: Grune & Stratton, 1977.

Romankiewicz, J. A., Gotz, V., Capelli, A., and Carlin, H. To improve patient adherence to drug regimens: An interdisciplinary approach. *American Journal of Nursing, 78,* 1216-1219, 1978.

Sanders, J. B., and Kardinal, C. G. Adaptive coping mechanisms in adult leukemia patients in remission. *Journal of the American Medical Association, 238,* 952-954, 1977.

Schmitt, F. E., and Wooldridge, P. J. Psychological preparation of surgical patients. *Nursing Research, 22,* 108-116, 1973.

Uustal, D. B. Values clarification in nursing. *American Journal of Nursing, 78,* 2058-2063, 1978.

Wright, B. A. *Physical Disability: A Psychological Approach.* New York: Harper & Row, Pubs. Inc., 1960.

Yura, H., and Walsh, M. B. *The Nursing Process: Assessing, Planning, Implementing, Evaluating.* New York: Appleton-Century-Crofts, 1973.

Chapter 12

COPING WITH CHILDHOOD CANCER: PROFESSIONAL AND FAMILY COMMUNICATION PATTERNS

John J. Spinetta* and Patricia M. Deasy

As with every child, so too with the child with cancer, the family is the primary environment through whose support the child is expected to grow into a happy and functional adult. Further, just as with every child, so too with the child with cancer, parents share a portion of their childrearing responsibilities with the educational system. The school, with its teachers, counselors, administrators, same-age-group peers, and rules and regulations is the supplementary environment through whose support and training the child is aided in his growth into a happy and functional adult. Because children reside within families, and because children attend school as the main workaday function of their young lives, our discussion of communication between the health care professional and the child with cancer will take into account the child's dependence upon family and school. In our discussion of the child with cancer, we will take the position of van Eys (1977) that the health care setting of the child with cancer is as much the family and the school as it is the hospital and clinic.

This chapter will focus on communication patterns between professionals in the health care setting and the child in his two essential growth environments: The family and the school. The chapter will be divided into the following sections:

---

*Portions of this chapter appear, in less detailed form, in J. Spinetta, "Disease-related Communication: How to Tell," in J. Kellerman (Ed.), Psychological Aspects of Childhood Cancer. Springfield: Thomas, 1979. The sections on family and school have been added and the chapter expanded and applied to the topic of this edited volume.

(a) Prerequisites to communicating with a child about his terminal illness,
(b) Communication patterns among family members;
(c) Communication between the health care professional and the family;
(d) Communication between the health care professional and the school.

PREREQUISITES TO COMMUNICATING WITH A CHILD ABOUT HIS TERMINAL ILLNESS

How does one communicate with a child about a potentially fatal illness? How does one talk to a child with cancer about the diagnosis, prognosis, and treatment regimen? Both parents and professionals alike find themselves in a dilemma. Adults often try to spare children the necessity of facing adult-like tasks before their time; yet avoiding the topic of death becomes increasingly difficult when the child has been diagnosed with a life-threatening illness. When the changes in the emotional climate surrounding the child become so obvious that the child senses that something very serious is wrong (Spinetta, 1974), it becomes necessary to deal honestly with the child's questions at the child's level of understanding. With the changed perspective in recent years regarding the lifespan of many children with cancer, the health care professional tends to respond to the child's questions early in the diagnosis with a reality-based hope and optimism, and parents are encouraged to keep their own hopes very much alive (Clapp, 1976; Koocher & Sallan, 1978; Lansky & Lowman, 1974; Van Eys, 1977). Yet the potential threat to life remains ever present, and one cannot hide the truth for very long. Whether told or not, the child will learn very quickly that he or she has cancer or leukemia and learn eventually that the disease is potentially fatal (Bluebond-Langner, 1974, 1977; Spinetta, 1974).

While hope of cure must be maintained, it would be unrealistic to think that a child over six years of age can be protected indefinitely from awareness of the potential fatality of the illness. Open use of the terms "cancer" and "leukemia" from the start, even with young children, will not necessarily lead to depression (Kellerman, Rigler, Siegel, & Katz, 1977); on the contrary, avoidance of the terms "cancer" and "leukemia" may compound the problem and lead to isolation and distrust when the child eventually discovers that the adults in his environment have been deceiving him (Spinetta, Rigler, & Karon, 1974). It is our own distinct belief and conviction that it is far better to address the issue of the seriousness of the child's illness from the very beginning (Spinetta, 1977, 1979). The task of telling a child about his diagnosis, treatment regimen, and potentially shortened life span is not an easy one, and certainly cannot be accomplished bluntly and in a single statement. While we stress the need for open and honest communication, the issues remain complex and very much related to the child's level of development. This section of the chapter will address prerequisites to communicating with a child about the illness. When one writes a "How to. . ." treatise, statements inevitably become prescriptive and subjective. The author makes no apologies for either. What is presented here is an approach to communication with the child based on a decade of both rigorous research and clinical practice in this area (Spinetta, 1979). The prerequisites discussed here apply throughout all sections of this chapter. Understanding the prerequisites is essential before one can undertake the stress-related task of communicating with the child about the illness.

The five prerequisites are:
 (1) The Parental Stance on Death: Philosophical Position;
 (2) The Parental Stance on Death: Emotional Position;
 (3) The Child's Age, Experience, and Level of Development;
 (4) Family Coping Strategies; and
 (5) The Child's Affinity for Process over Content.

The Parental Stance on Death: Philosophical Position

An essential prerequisite to communication with the child about his or her illness is a basic understanding of the family's view of life (Kantor & Lehr, 1975; Lewis, Beavers, Gossett & Phillips, 1976). It is especially important when dealing with an issue so basic to the human condition as a potential threat to life that one understand both the force of the basic parenting demand (Sheposh, Spinetta,

Chadwick and Elliott, 1978), and the critical role of the family as the prime emotional and intellectual environment for the child (Spinetta & Maloney, 1978). A family resides within a larger social and cultural context, both intrafamilial and extrafamilial. A family has a manner of facing life, a manner of placing meaning to the mystery of life and death, that may be long-standing within the traditions of past generations; or of brief standing within the context of a new-found cosmology; or even lacking altogether, for want of ever having had the need or courage to face the issue previously (Toynbee, 1976). This social context of the family's private cosmology/theology/philosophy of life and death is the environment from which the child will draw his or her own meaning and strength. It is necessary that the professionals both understand the parent's philosophy of life and also come to terms with their own view of the purpose of life and death. Should there be a discrepancy between the professional's view and the parent's view, it is not advisable for the professional to attempt to change the parent's beliefs at this time. To attempt to replace the parental cosmology at so critical a time as the crisis point of diagnosis of cancer can lead to ultimate failure in coping and adaptation for the child while he is alive (Spinetta, 1978, Spinetta & Maloney, 1978), and most especially to a failure in ultimate adaptation of the parents and surviving siblings after the death of the child. In a recent study (Spinetta, Swarner, Kard & Sheposh, 1978), it was demonstrated that firm commitment to a family-consistent and time-honored view of the place of death in life was critical to the ultimate adaptive efforts of the surviving family members.

In brief, professionals who talk to the child must keep in mind that families differ in what they bring to the illness in terms of philosophical stance on the place of death in life. The professional must guide the family in its efforts to tap its own basic strengths, rather than attempt at this critical time to pursue a course of radical change in the parental views.

The Parental Stance on Death: Emotional Position

As important as the parental cosmology is to the family's ultimate adaptive efforts, even more important is how well the family has incorporated that stance (Glock, 1965). It is not so much what death is that concerns most of us; it is rather how we feel about death (Feifel, 1977; Jackson, 1965; Kastenbaum, 1977). When one is dealing with the parents of a child who has been diagnosed with a life-threatening illness it is critical to be patient and to allow time to become aware of, and help the parents become aware of, both their general and their specific attitudes and emotional responses toward the concept of death. Has the family experienced death before? Was it a grandparent; an uncle or aunt; a close friend or neighbor? What was the mother's reaction? What was the father's reaction? Did they grieve at the same pace or in different manners? Did they share their feelings of grief with each other and with other family members, or did they suffer in isolation and silence. Did they involve the children? At what age? Knowledge of the general and specific history of the family's emotional approach to the concept of death is the second prerequisite to talking to the child about his own potentially life-threatening illness.

The Child's Age, Experience, and Level of Development

A third prerequisite to communication with a child about his illness is a basic understanding of developmental levels in the growth of the child's thought processes, notably those surrounding the concepts of life and death. There are many books and articles which speak to this issue (for example, Easson, 1970; Grollman, 1967; Hostler, 1978; Jackson, 1965; Spinetta, Spinetta, Kung & Schwartz, 1976). Although it is difficult to do justice to so complex a topic in so brief a space, we will address this issue at this point in an overview fashion, so that we can place the issue in proper perspective. We will address the topic in two phases: (1) the healthy child and death, and (2) the seriously ill child and death.

The Healthy Child and Death

Concepts of death are age-related in children and differ with intellectual ability and development (Spinetta, Spinetta, Kung & Schwartz, 1976). It is generally believed that during the first two years of life, there is no understanding of death as such, but fear of separation from protecting, conforting persons is present in its most terrifying intensity. While death is not yet a fact of life for the child going on three, anxiety about separation remains all pervasive. Some time between the ages of three and five, most children first comprehend the fact of death as something that happens to others. At this time, the concept of death is still vague. It is associated with sleep and the absence of light or movement and is not yet thought of as permanent. In contrast to toddlers, most children of this age are able to withstand and understand short separation. They often respond more spontaneously and with less anxiety to questions about death than do older children. They are also curious about dead animals and flowers. However, children between three and five typically deny death as a final reality. They believe death is accidental and they themselves will not die. (Aradine, 1976).

Attitudes and concepts of children do not change abruptly at any given age, but evolve gradually and with wide individual variation. This is true whether one is talking about the concept of time, the concept of space, or the concept of death. From approximately the age of six onward, the child seems gradually to be accommodating himself or herself to the proposition that death is final, inevitable, universal and personal. Many six and seven year-olds suspect that their parents will die some day and that they too may die, but only in the very distant future. Children in these early school years show a strong tendency to personify death. Many children at their initial awareness and discovery of death are horrified, confused, and angered. Although some recent authors feel that a child in the present day and age is coming to grips with the concept of death at a younger age than ever before because of exposure (Hansen, 1973), most still agree that the child under ten has not yet attained a well-developed understanding of death. As children approach adolescence, they are equipped with the intellectual tools necessary to understand time, space, life, and death in a logical manner. At about the age of ten or eleven the fact of the universality and the permanence of death becomes understandable.

What we have discussed to this point is the normal development of the ability to conceptualize in the healthy child. A speeding up of the process occurs when the child is faced with death at an early age, at a level preceding the ability to conceptualize it (Bluebond-Langner, 1974, 1977; Spinetta, 1974).

The Seriously Ill Child and Death

How does all this apply to the child who has been diagnosed with a potentially life-threatening illness? Recent studies of six-to-ten year-old leukemic children reveal that, despite efforts by parents and medical personnel to keep the child from becoming aware of the prognosis, he somehow picks up a sense that the illness is no ordinary illness. The fear of abandonment and separation, characteristic of the younger child, has added to it a fear of bodily harm and injury and possible awareness of his own impending death, or, at the very least, the awareness at a level preceding his ability to conceptualize it, that something very serious is happening. The awareness of one's own impending death becomes stronger as the child nears death (Bluebond-Langner, 1974, 1977; Spinetta, Rigler & Karon, 1973, 1974).

Despite the great efforts often expended on the part of physicians and parents to protect the young children from awareness of the prognosis, the children can and do become aware of the seriousness of their illness, at an age much younger than such awareness occurs in their healthy counterparts.

It is important, then, in speaking with children with cancer about the concept of death, to understand differences in ability to conceptualize that are due to the child's age and level of development, but at the same time, to keep in mind that a child who is experiencing the cancer and the often drastic changes in the emotional climate around him often becomes aware of his own impending demise at a much younger age than his healthy peers and at a level that often the child himself cannot conceptualize.

Family Coping Strategies

A fourth prerequisite to communication with a child about the potentially fatal nature of the cancer is an understanding of the family's usual manner of dealing with crises. An understanding of the past, present, and possibly changing coping modes of the various family members as individuals, and of the family as a social group is essential if a professional is to tap the family's own resource pool. Individuals have different levels of stress tolerance, different levels of ability to deal with stress, different histories of success and failure in overcoming stress (Selye, 1974, 1976). What works for the professional may not work at all for the family, especially when the family is in the middle of sustaining the burden of the diagnosis of cancer in their child. The very diagnosis itself can shift the family's central survival skills to a newer mode. At this stage in the family's development, the individual members need a professional who is willing to understand and help them strengthen their usual mode of coping with crises, help them grow into facing this crisis, give them the tolerance and patience they will need to make the transition, and remain noncritical in the process. This is not a time for imposition. It is a time for support.

The Child's Affinity for Process over Content

The fifth and final prerequisite for communicating with a child about the potential threat to his own life is a basic understanding of how a child works. In this author's experience, it is more important to know how to talk about the death process than it is to know what to say (content). At a level long preceding the ability to verbalize, a young infant can pick up subtle and not-so-subtle cues of tension, anger, or happiness from the mother. As children grow, they remain very much attuned to nonverbal cues in their environment (Mussen, Conger & Kagan; 1974). They are very dependent on the adults around them to help explain to them what they are feeling. In a warm and close family, the parents will try to explain to the child what he or she is feeling and soothe the child's expressed concerns. However, when the parents reach an area that may be of some emotional distress for them as adults, such as the area of potential threat to life, they may fall short of their usual attempts at explanation. If children do not find a real explanation to fit what they sense, they may let their imaginations take over. They may assume that they did something wrong, and that's why mommy and daddy won't explain this to them. They may feel that the medical intrusions are punishments for wrongdoing. Unless the parents explain to the child, at his or her level, what is happening, the child may have to deal with imagined fears, distresses, and concerns that are much more disturbing and difficult to deal with than the actual facts.

Children are attuned to nonverbal cues in their environment. An understanding of this concept is a prerequisite to meaningful communication with the child.

COMMUNICATION PATTERNS AMONG FAMILY MEMBERS

It seems clear from recent studies that the fatally ill child over six years of age is concerned about his illness, and that even though this concern may not always take the form of overt expressions about his impending death, the more subtle fears and anxieties are nonetheless real, painful, and very much related to the seriousness of the illness that the child is experiencing. Whether or not one wishes to call this unconceptualized anxiety of the child about his own fatal illness "death anxiety" seems to be a problem of semantics rather than of fact. The fatally ill child reacts to the illness in a manner exhibiting a much greater anxiety than his chronically, but not fatally, ill counterpart. This awareness is present, regardless of whether or not the family wishes the child to know. The children eventually come to an awareness of the seriousness of their illness (Bluebond-Langner, 1974, 1977; Spinetta, 1974; and Waechter, 1971).

If it is true that a child as young as six is aware of the serious nature of his or her illness, what does the child do with this knowledge and awareness? Does the child talk openly with his family about the prognosis, or does the child live in silence with the knowledge? What role does the family play in the child's wishing to talk or not to talk about the illness? To help answer these questions, Spinetta and Maloney (1978) studied family communication patterns around the issue of cancer in the child. Results showed that the level of family communication about the illness, as expressed in the mothers' judgment of communication, was related to coping strategies in the child. Families in which levels of communication about the illness were high were those families in which the children: (1) exhibited a nondefensive personal posture, (2) expressed a consistently close relationship with the parents, and (3) expressed a basic satisfaction with self.

The child who has the personal desire and parental permission to discuss his illness openly within the family structure is in the best position to receive the type of support he most needs (Spinetta, 1978).

Circumstances of pain, reactions to medication and treatment, and the death of other children from the illness, all play a role in the child's increasing awareness of the severity of his or her illness. But above all, the parental level of willingness to discuss the illness is critical to the child's decision about what to do with the knowledge. There are those professionals who would encourage denial in order for the children to maintain mental as well as physical comfort, and up to a point, some denial may be effective (Alby & Alby, 1973; Howarth, 1974). But the evidence is beginning to mount that the children, siblings, and parents would be best served by being encouraged to bring into the open their anxieties about the illness and its possible consequences (Bluebond-Langner, 1974, 1977; Futterman & Hoffman, 1973; Spinetta, Spinetta, Kung & Schwartz, 1976).

Spinetta, Swarner, et al., 1979, conducted a series of interviews with families whose children had died of cancer. The most frequently discussed issue with families whose children were over six at the time of death was the extent to which the family had communicated with the child about the possible terminal effects of the illness. Of the families interviewed, about half felt they had talked freely and openly with their young child about his or her impending death. None of the parents who had spoken openly with their young child felt that too much had been said; on the contrary, the parents felt that a higher level of closeness was achieved with the child than might have occurred otherwise. The memory of the open discussions and exchange of family values before the child's death had sustained the families during the mourning process. The siblings in the open group reported having had time to say goodbye to their dying brother or sister, to resolve old quarrels, and to help the dying child in his or her own efforts to say goodbye as well.

In contrast, of those families whose child had died without open discussion of the illness or of the imminent death, the majority reported wishing that they had spoken more openly with the child. The parents reported feelings of incompleteness and nonresolution. Those siblings who reported unresolved feelings regretted not having been forewarned or not having had time to say goodbye and settle differences before the child's death.

In brief, the children with cancer were found to resolve the issues surrounding their diagnosis, treatment, and prognosis more effectively when allowed to speak openly about the cancer. Mothers, fathers, and siblings reported in postdeath interviews that resolution of the grief process was facilitated by their memories of having done all they could for their child, most notably by openness in levels of communication about the illness.

Certainly, further research is called for and further guidelines must be sought regarding what to say and when, taking into consideration the severity of the illness, parental and sibling readiness, and age levels of the children. Nevertheless, studies to date point to the fact that the child already knows, at some level, that the illness is serious. Allowing the child to talk about the illness can have generally beneficial short- and long-term effects on all family members, including the life-threatened child.

A word of caution is appropriate lest the statements be interpreted as a blanket support for open communication in all families in all circumstances. Although we are pointing to the generally supportive value to the sick child of open patterns of family communication, a forced openness too soon for some families can be destructive. There are parents who demonstrate a marked inability to function under the stress and others who exhibit maladaptive behavior, becoming inaccessible, withdrawn, and remote (Futterman, Hoffman & Sabshin, 1972; Koupernik, 1973; Spinetta, Spinetta, Kung & Schwartz, 1976; Willis, 1974). The goal in working with such families must be to help the family members eventually become aware of the false sense of equilibrium that may come from an excessive denial of the problem, and the harm such denial can cause the sick child. If a temporary use of denial, especially at the beginning, proves helpful in allowing the family time to pull together adaptive resources, then such short-lived denial can be useful in the overall adaptive effort.

It is our theory that the fatally ill child chooses whether or not to talk about his illness based on past and present experience within the family regarding openness of communication about the illness. The child may choose silence because he is aware, even at a level preceding his ability to express it, that his family does not allow communication about the illness. Or the child may choose to communicate honestly about the illness because of a family history reinforcing openness, and because he is supported by present parental attitudes. Each choice may be viewed as a different style of coping. The choice for silence can lead to excessive denial and avoidance, place distance between the child and his sources of support, and lead to a feeling of rejection and isolation and to the child's awareness of being left alone to work out his or her problems. Such a feeling of rejection and isolation comes from a level of denial supported and encouraged within the child's family. A forced openness in such a family might appear to the child as an even worse alternative than his suffering in silence. In contrast, a choice for open discussion, stemming from the sincere attempts of family members to communicate concern and support allows overt expression of feelings. Such expressions of a child's fears relative to the illness, deriving from openness in levels of family communication can at the child's own request lead to mutual support among family members helping the child achieve a balanced adaptive equilibrium.

Closed communication about the illness may appear on the surface to be the simplest solution to the question of how some family members may deal with the childhood cancer—denial of a problem makes it go away, for a while. But the fatally ill child in such a family expresses unhappiness, alienation, and feelings of being left alone to work out his or her fate. In contrast, opening up levels of communication within the family is like opening the proverbial Pandora's box. A complex set of feelings emerges. Openness increases expressed levels of anxiety within the family and commits family members, as well as all others who must deal with the family members, to a confrontation with the severity of the illness. The open family may be torn apart by the confrontation or it may come through the adaptive struggle with members having grown closer together, having gained a mature ability to struggle valiantly in future life conflicts, and having achieved a level of confidence, strength, and reevaluation of basic life commitments that will make for a more effective and fulfilled life.

In discussing the concept of coping, it must be kept in mind that everyone copes. Whether well or poorly, people make it through a crisis (Lazarus & Launier, 1978). Even escape through suicide or mental illness is a functional manner of dealing with a crisis situation. The person is coping in a manner that is socially maladapted, but is nonetheless coping. In our discussion of individuals coping with cancer, it is important to place the coping patterns of the child, sibling, mother, or father within the context of the family in its primary role as support environment for its members. If we find a family in which there is a loss of common objectives, a reduction in cooperation among family members, withholding of reciprocity of services (most notably in the sexual roles of the spouses), lack of coordination of functions, and lack of consensus of emotional attitudes, then, no matter how well an individual member may seem to be adapting to the diagnosis of cancer in a member of the family, the family itself has failed in its primary function of social support of its members. The result is family disorganization at the least, and possible family disintegration if the situation continues for long. Although Lansky, Cairns, Hassanein, Wehr & Lowman (1978) have shown that families of children with cancer do not separate or divorce as frequently as families of children with emotional problems, the families do disintegrate at levels of frequency much higher than that of nonstressed families. Thus, while individual family members may cope effectively and well without family support, what we have found in recent studies is that such effective coping is the exception in families in which communication is minimal and disorganization is high.

In the family of a child with cancer, parents are often so overwhelmed by the sickness itself that they do not make adequate preparations for ordinary events. Thus a child diagnosed with leukemia at two years of age can at six years of age begin to have problems in school simply because the mother does not engage in the ordinary maternal preparatory steps to school. An event such as the child's entering first grade is so minor in the mother's eyes, in comparison with the illness itself, that the mother does not hear the child's plea for help or tend to the child's needs. Had the child not been diagnosed with cancer three years previously, the mother would have placed into perspective the child's true needs for preparation for first grade, with its accompanying social demands from the child's school-aged peers. What has happened is a basic failure in family communication, because the mother's attempts at coping with her child's illness, though successful regarding the illness, leave the mother with little energy to deal with the child's new problem, entry into school. The mother is coping with the cancer but is not giving her child the type of family support the child needs in his or her own coping efforts in a nondisease task. In like manner, ordinary life transitions of children, such as entry into junior high school, pubescence, or transfer to a new city, can take on crisis proportions because the family, overwhelmed by the diagnosis of cancer in the child, has frozen efforts at growth. It is as if the family unit were saying to itself: "If only we can hold it all together and keep from falling apart, we'll make it." Such a mode of coping with the cancer precludes the type of openness to growth and changes that is necessary as the children move through various developmental crises on their way to adulthood. Such a family fails to give the necessary energy in helping the child in his or her time of greatest nondisease need.

What has been stated about the child with cancer holds even more so for the siblings. The siblings of children with cancer are often neglected by the parents, not because their needs are not important, but because their needs take on a lesser importance relative to the seriousness of the diagnosis of cancer. Siblings in the families of the children with cancer often find themselves facing all alone, without parental support, developmental tasks that are overwhelming when faced alone. Attempts by the siblings to seek help from parents are often met, not with resistance, but with a plea to the siblings to be mature and generous and respect the needs of the ill child. Even the mentally strong and healthy sibling cannot be expected to go through life's transitional stages with little or no support from parents who have already "burned out" from strategies used in coping with their ill child's diagnosis.

Finally, what has been stated about the child with cancer and the siblings holds as much for the parents as for the children. The parents, often in unison but more frequently in their own separate ways, expend their energies in dealing with the cancer. What typically happens is that the remainder of their life tasks, such as career, finances, and sexual life, take on a lowered significance. When the spouse's needs are unmet within the family unit, the spouse must perforce turn outside the family to fulfill the needs.

In brief, a family expends an inordinate amount of energy in attempts to keep itself from disorganization and disintegration under the overwhelming threat to the life of one of its members. In the process of dealing with the cancer, the family as a unit finds itself with little energy or direction left in fulfilling its primary function as a support system to each of its members. Individual members, who have needs that go far beyond that of dealing with the diagnosis of cancer, find these needs unmet. What is called for is a communication of these needs at a level that can be effectively understood by other members of the family. Unless this communication is consistent and clear, and unless each family member is allowed to continue receiving support even for so-called "minor" needs from the family system, that individual will be forced to look elsewhere for the type of support the family is no longer giving.

The goal of work with the families of children with cancer must be to help them strengthen the adaptive capabilities and coping styles specific to that family. The professional in the health care setting who is attempting to treat the child for the cancer must take into account the family structure and environment in which the child finds himself, if that professional is truly interested in a "totally cured child" (van Eys, 1977). To help the family members struggle forward as best they can in a commitment to the value of the remaining months or years of their child's life, and to give them access to the intrafamilial and extrafamilial sources of support they will need to help them, both in the struggle and in the grieving after the child's death, becomes an all-encompassing goal which the professional in the health care setting must strive for if he or she has as a goal not only the care of the child's illness, but the care of the total child. The generally beneficial effects of open communication on family members, and above all, on the life-threatened child, has been demonstrated. What needs to be discussed at this point is what the professional in the health care setting can do to facilitate functional levels of open communication within the family. This issue will be addressed in the following section of the chapter.

COMMUNICATION BETWEEN THE HEALTH CARE PROFESSIONALS AND THE FAMILY

It is understandable that the experienced professional has had and will continue to have reasonable objections to talking to a child about the seriousness of his or her illness. There are common objections to talking to a child with cancer about his possible impending death (Spinetta, 1979). We will state these objections and then attempt to respond to the objections with data from research studies. Eight objections will be discussed in logical order.

OBJECTION ONE. The child does not know about death, let alone his own possible impending death. We should not add to his burden by telling him things that he may not even imagine.

RESPONSE ONE. The child does know, at an age much younger than we have previously imagined (Bluebond-Langner, 1974, 1977; Spinetta, Rigler & Karon, 1973, 1974). By talking to the child about the possibility of his own early death, one is not telling him anything new; one is merely giving him permission to speak freely of his concerns. Several years ago, when the medical care for childhood cancer was in its infancy, the diagnosis of cancer in the child was typically followed very shortly by death. Many physicians at that time felt that the child should be protected from knowledge of the fatality of the illness. As medical progress has increased the survival rate of the child with cancer, this increased life span has brought with it a change of attitudes toward communicating with the child about the illness. The great majority of professionals dealing with children with cancer now advocate an open and honest approach with the child in the manner suggested above.

OBJECTION TWO. If it is true that one is confirming the child's suspicions then it would seem clear that even if the child suspects, he is better off not being told outright.

RESPONSE TWO. The fear of the unknown is worse than the fear of the known, most especially in a child (Kastenbaum, 1977; Mussen, et al. 1974). The child who is not allowed to share becomes isolated, depressed, and filled with confusion (Spinetta, 1974; Spinetta & Maloney, 1975, 1978).

OBJECTION THREE. Communicating with the child will not help him; it will only open up a Pandora's box that had best be left alone. The adults in the child's world have the strength necessary to shoulder the burden and it is not fair to force the child to share such a burden at so young an age.

RESPONSE THREE. Communication reduces feelings of isolation, self-dislike and despair (Spinetta & Maloney, 1978). Allowing the child a chance to express concerns, both negative and positive, eventually leads that child to a healthier self-concept and to the ability to live as normal a life and as full a life as possible within the context of the illness.

OBJECTION FOUR. Communication will hurt the siblings and parents in the long run because they will have to live with the knowledge that they failed to protect their young child from the burden of awareness.

RESPONSE FOUR. Communication is best for the parents in the long run (Binger, Ablin, et al., 1969; Futterman & Hoffman, 1973; Hofer, Wolff, Friedman, & Mason, 1972; Spinetta & Spinetta, 1979; Spinetta, Swarner, Kard & Sheposh, 1978; and Stehbens & Lascari, 1974). Those parents interviewed one full year after the death of their child, who showed the healthiest and most advanced level of adaptation to life without their child, were those parents who reported having spent the years of the diagnosis and illness communicating openly with their child upon request (Spinetta, Swarner, Kard & Sheposh, 1978) and in a manner appropriate to the child's age and developmental level.

OBJECTION FIVE. Talking about a potentially shortened life span with your own child may prove harmful to other parents and children who, for example, may overhear you talking in a hospital waiting room. You must be sensitive to the needs of others.

RESPONSE FIVE. It helps other parents to talk about it, to get their feelings out in the open. It also reduces tension and allows the families to be prepared for untoward eventualities (Spinetta, Spinetta, Kung & Schwartz, 1976; Townes, Wold & Holmes, 1974).

OBJECTION SIX. Not all families can endure or sustain such levels of openness. You must be sensitive to the needs and abilities and levels of readiness of specific families.

RESPONSE SIX. This is very true, as stated above. While families cannot be categorized into types, our research (Spinetta 1977, 1978) has shown that there are at least three family approaches to the issue of communication and support: (1) supportive, (2) quasi-supportive, and (3) noncommunicative. There are some families who, because of a past history of dealing with crises, or because of personality, philosophy, and basic view of life not only talk openly within their family about life's concerns, but allow their children and themselves the freedom to openly express both positive and negative feelings. Such families prove themselves most supportive to the needs of individual members. Other families, those we term quasi-supportive, may talk openly about the illness, but seem to fall short of allowing the child and other family members, including themselves, to talk openly about feelings, both positive and negative. In such families, there is often a nonmalicious, well-intentioned resistance to open communication that forces the levels of support underground. In some such families, the levels of support may be less than genuine (Spinetta, 1978). Finally, there are those families we term noncommunicative, that openly admit to not being able to even mention the word cancer, and who do not allow conversation either about death or about other crises in the family structure. While such families may appear to need greater levels of communication, it is critical to allow such families the time and room to move forward at their own pace in dealing with their response to illness.

OBJECTION SEVEN. If I, as a professional in the hospital structure, take the time out of my busy medical day to discuss with a family the psychosocial issues surrounding the prognosis, then I have opened up a new plateau of communication with that family. I will no longer be able to deal solely with the medical. I will be forced to deal with problems at the more time-consuming level of the psychosocial. I cannot deal with all of my other patients in this way. I am not trained to handle such problems. It would be unfair to try to do so.

RESPONSE SEVEN. This is a very true point. It is becoming more and more difficult for physicians to treat the child without becoming increasingly involved in the inner workings of the family. The physicians find themselves becoming more involved with the families whose child is being treated for cancer. Medical decisions for continued chemotherapy or additional surgery are becoming increasingly conjoint decisions between physician and parent. As the atmosphere of open communication begins to take hold, the physicians find themselves becoming involved in psychosocial areas of concern for which many if not most have been ill-trained. Alby & Alby (1973) spoke to this issue when they discussed the necessity of having a "psy-person" on each team dealing with childhood cancer. It is often unfair to the doctors to demand that they take the effort to deal with the family's psychosocial problems; it is unfair to the family to have a physician not trained in the psychosocial or unwilling to do so, attempt to deal in a haphazard manner with the problem. Some physicians in institutional settings may have the time to deal with such problems and may wish to do so with certain families. However, in many institutions, it may be reasonable to assign a person with psychological expertise, when finances and institutional agreements permit, to deal with such issues.

OBJECTION EIGHT. I can't take it. I'll burn out. There is no way that I, as a professional dealing with these areas, can continue to deal at an intense personal and familial level, on a daily basis, and keep giving of myself at this level over time. I cannot continue doing this without being affected.

RESPONSE EIGHT. Very true. What is becoming a serious problem for the physicians has been a long-standing problem for the nonmedical professionals in the health care setting who have been dealing directly with the psychosocial issues surrounding the diagnosis of cancer in the child. This is an area of intense stress-related transactions (Lazarus & Launier, 1978). There really is no way that a professional in the health care setting—physician, nurse, psychologist, social worker, or minister—can continue to respond to the needs of families, parents, children, siblings, fellow staff members, and oneself continually over time, without burning out (Axlerod, 1978; Schowalter, 1978; Viles, 1978). There are several solutions to the problem: (1) Remove oneself from the feeling level. Deal with the children as objects to be studied and cured. (2) Give totally and completely to each family that demands it; burn out early, leave the profession. (3) Deal with burn-out before it occurs. This can be accomplished by: (a) talking to one's medical peers about the problems that occur in working with families at this close a level, and (b) learning to "get away." Getting away could mean taking long weekends off, days off, vacations, or learning to reduce levels of stress by a variety of self-relaxation techniques now in vogue (Lecron, 1964; Selye, 1974, 1976).

There is, then, a decreasing need to convince physicians and other health care professionals dealing with the child with cancer of the need for open and honest communication with the child. What is appearing now is the issue of the manner in which to communicate with the child and family. What professionals in the health care setting are now asking with increasing frequency is: how do I talk to the family? What do I say about the potentially shortened life span of the child? How do I approach the child and when?

As we have noted above, there are five prerequisites to talking to a child about his or her own potentially shortened life span. Critical factors for the professional include not only becoming aware of the child's level of development, the familial patterns and coping strategies, and the family's attitudes toward death, but above all must include the professional's awareness of his or her own philosophic and emotional position toward the place of death in his or her own life. While this task of facing one's own death may be impossible to fulfill in its entirety (Sahler, 1978), at least an initial attempt at self-awareness is critical before one undertakes to communicate with a family about the child's diagnosis, treatment, and prognosis.

An awareness of family dynamics, as outlined in the third section of this chapter, is also critical for any health care professional who wishes to effectively aid the family in its concerns. Once one has begun the task of mastery of all of the above at least in an initial fashion, one is ready to begin communicating with the families about their child. The specific content of the communication will be determined by the individual circumstances surrounding the medical condition, and the specific family dynamics involved. Such must remain the judgment of the professional in each task. It is the communication process that forms the main tenet of this chapter.

Whatever can be done to facilitate understanding in the family, whatever can be done to convince the family of the need to keep open the channels of communication within the family and between the family and hospital, should be attempted. Various authors stress the use of parent groups, explanatory handbooks, continued responses to direct questions of parents and children, availability of the professional caregiver, and use of techniques of self-relaxation, such as hypnosis. The main point is to be open with one's self to the family. Be prepared with prerequisites. Then keep all channels of communication open (Spinetta, Spinetta, Kung & Schwartz, 1976).

HOW TO TALK TO A CHILD ABOUT DEATH

Now that we have dealt with prerequisites and addressed several objections to communication with the child about the potential fatality of the illness, what are our suggestions about the process of talking to the child about death? The following points are suggested as topics to be raised with a child, in an age-appropriate manner, at the child's own level of readiness. It is important to keep in mind the prerequisites mentioned above, and to place the conversation within the context of the specific and personal environmental history of the child, in the specific familial and institutional environment.

In the author's own experience, the following points have proved beneficial to the child, when couched in the child's own language, and raised in a tactful process-oriented manner (Spinetta, 1979). Some of the points may be raised at the child's initial expression of concern over a possibly impending death. Others are best reserved for the child whose disease course has brought him very close to the actual point of death. In all cases, it is important to remain aware of the child's level of concern. The author has found it helpful to explain to the child that:

(1) Death is a part of the natural order of things. It happens sooner for some, later for others. The child's disease may shorten his life span, but we do not know how much. It is good to keep hope alive.

(2) Death has a social significance. We have special feelings for the other persons we share our lives with, as they do for us.
(3) Death is a separation on both sides. Not only does the person who dies lose the people left behind, but they lose their child as well.
(4) The loss is never complete. The deceased lives on in some way. (Here the specific cosmological stance of the family is critical; some feel that the child will live on in spirit; others that the child will have passed on a legacy of the meaning of life to friends; and others that the child will live on in both body and soul for eternity.)
(5) The child will not be alone at death and after. (What the child is looking for is parental presence and support throughout, both during the death process and after death. It is important to reassure these children that they will not be suffering death alone, and that the parents will remain with them even after death. This last point is critical, essential to the child, and of necessity to be phrased within the context of the parent's cosmological stance, as with point 4.
(6) At the point of death, people, whether adults or children, have the need to know that they have done all that they could with life. This is a universal human concern that is shared by children as well as by adults. Even young children can live fulfilled and happy lives before they die. It is not necessary to live to eighty-five to make a lasting contribution to the human condition. Young children can touch the minds and hearts of those they deal with at school, in the hospital, at home, in a manner that will live on in others' memories. If the child's life, manner of facing the illness, and death can help modify a parent's, sibling's, or professional's attitude in a manner that helps move the human condition one step further forward, that child will have contributed to humanity and will have led a highly effective life in a short period of time.
(7) It's all right to cry and to feel sad. The feelings of sadness will come and go. The child will often feel sad when he thinks about his illness.

(8) It's all right to feel angry and resentful. The feelings of anger will come and go, too.
(9) It's all right not to want to talk to anyone anymore about it for a while. We can't keep talking about death all the time. Sometimes it is best to tell parents or friends that you don't want to talk about it now.
(10) When the child is ready to talk about it, the adult will be there to listen and support. (This had better be true.)
(11) It is not necessary to express how you feel in words. Sometimes it's all right just to sit there and not have to talk. And if what you say when you want to talk sounds confused or silly, that's all right too. Adults don't always know what to say either.
(12) When it finally comes, death will not hurt. The dying process may be painful, and the doctor will do all that can be done to reduce the pain to a minimum, but death itself won't hurt. The pain will never return again. (Children are very concerned with having the pain finally end. It is important to reassure them that it will finally end.)
(13) When someone that we love dies, it is important to be able to say goodbye. People have a social custom of saying their last goodbyes together, crying together, talking over what is happening. Sometimes, the person who is going to die will want to call his friends in to say goodbye. This is a very good thing to do. It makes him feel better and makes his friends, brothers and sisters, and parents feel better, too. Afterwards, his mother and father will want to have their friends over, too, to talk about him and how much they love him. Sometimes the adults do this in the privacy of their homes; sometimes they do it in church. These goodbye group-happenings are usually called funerals. They are very important for the child's mother and father, and brothers and sisters.
(14) Grown-ups sometimes don't know very much about death either. If parents talk with a doctor and cry afterwards, or if they talk about their child's illness and become teary-eyed, it's because they love their child and don't want to lose him. However, if a child has to die, his parents, family and

friends will remember the happy times, and the child's memory will live on in mind and spirit. (See numbers 4 and 5 above.) Parents are happy knowing their children have been happy.

The above points are highly subjective and are listed here because they have proved helpful in the past in the author's conversations with children (Spinetta, 1979). They remain suggestions to be applied with caution and judgment, at the child's own bidding, and at a level a child is comfortable with. The most important of all the suggestions and prescriptions listed above, to be kept in mind throughout any conversation with a child, is that a child is more process-oriented than content-oriented. Children pay less attention to what you say, and more to your concern, how you say what you are saying, and the body language you use when you are attempting to communicate your concerns and offers of help. Although the content of your communications is not unimportant, what you say is critical; you say all sorts of things and make all sorts of "mistakes" in what you say, and the child will overlook that, if your manner is in tune with the child. However, no matter how well rehearsed and "correct" your content is, if your manner is lacking or not in tune with the child, you may find that the conversation was in one direction only. It is important to keep in mind the time frame of the child. What is said early in the diagnosis period in response to the child's questions, will be more in a context of hope for lengthy survival. What is said near the point of death will be more along the lines of points 11-14.

How do you talk to children about their own possible early death from cancer? With great difficulty, with great concern, with care for the child, and with a heavy price on your own emotions and feelings. But the reward for your efforts will be a child who is able to face you in turn as a mature person, at whatever age and developmental level, and feel with you that he or she is not alone in facing the most difficult task any one of us has to face in our lives, the fact of our own death. The failure to make the attempt can only lead to isolation, loneliness, and ultimate despair in the child. Making the attempt, giving the child the social support and understanding most needed at that time, has as its reward the fullest gift we can share with the child with cancer: our own love, understanding, and shared concern for each of our roles in the basic human condition.

COMMUNICATION BETWEEN HEALTH CARE PROFESSIONALS AND THE SCHOOL

A major part of normal growth and development for all children, including the sick child, involves school. For a child with cancer a return to school represents a continuation of life, hope for the future, socialization with peers, and an attempt to reestablish equilibrium—an equilibrium that does not deny the fact of the cancer, but encompasses the new reality base of cancer.

Most pediatric hematology-oncology teams make great efforts to maintain good communication among the physician, nurse, social service personnel, parents, and child. As shown above, children with cancer, as young as six years of age, were found to resolve the issues surrounding their diagnosis, treatment, and prognosis more effectively when allowed to speak openly about the cancer (Spinetta, 1978). Children with cancer return to school with these awarenesses and their accompanying concerns. School personnel play a crucial role in determining whether or not the child with cancer can live a normal life, since so much of the child's day is centered around school. Teachers, counselors, school nurses, and administrators must be prepared to deal with this added responsibility.

A return to school for a child with cancer involves personal interaction with typically one teacher at the elementary school level, five or more at the secondary level, and the school nurse, counselor, and administrator, in addition to peers. Each person brings to the understanding of the child with cancer, her own philosophy of life, attitude toward death, and understanding of cancer (Spinetta, 1979). Furthermore, each school and each district often has a distinctively identifiable attitude toward working with any child with a medical problem in the regular classroom. It is, therefore, imperative to prepare significant school personnel for the reentry of the patient-student.

Since diagnosis, the child with cancer has received the best possible medical care from his physicians, and love and concern from his family. When he is considered medically ready to return to school, it is important to prepare the school environment to receive and nurture the child. Not to prepare the school adequately, the environment in which he spends an average of five to six hours per day, is to jeopardize the child's attempt to cope with his school life within the context of his diagnosis.

Preparing the Teacher

PHILOSOPHY OF DEATH. While individuals associated with the medical aspects of cancer realize that children with cancer are living longer, professionals outside this environment frequently equate cancer with death. Because this equation of cancer with death is not always accurate, this attitude must be addressed if teachers are to be adequately prepared. Just as each member of the medical staff has his own philosophical position on death, so too does each member of the school staff. A specific teacher's philosophy of death may differ from that of colleagues, and from that of the parents of the child with cancer. Nonetheless, the presence of a possibly life-threatened child in the classroom causes reflection and concern among the school staff. For some this can be a personally unsettling experience.

Not only do individual teachers have a personal philosophy of death, they also have an emotional position. How people feel about death is as important as how they think about it. Teachers have had different experiences with death, and each has had different means of coping with grief. It is important to assist teachers to become aware of both their general attitudes, and their specific attitudes, and their emotional responses toward the concept of death.

FAMILY COPING. While it is an important prerequisite for teachers to come to terms with their own philosophy and emotional stance on death, as well as gain an appreciation of the child's understanding of death at different ages, it is also as necessary for them, as for the physicians, to realize that each family has its own manner of dealing with crises. Individuals have different levels of stress tolerance, different levels of ability to deal with stress, different histories of success and failure in overcoming stress (Selye, 1974, 1976). The very diagnosis of cancer itself can shift the family's central survival skills to a newer mode (Spinetta, 1978). The teacher must realize that she is working not only with a child but also with a family in crisis.

When communicating with teachers it is important to help them realize that children, all children, and especially the children with cancer, are very sensitive to nonverbal cues in their environment. The child will sense at a nonverbal level if a teacher is uneasy about his presence in the classroom; he can also sense a warm, caring, supportive attitude.

IMPORTANCE OF HOPE. The emphasis to this point has been to help the teacher come to terms with his or her philosophy and emotional stance on death, understand children's developmental understanding of death, children's affinity for process over content, as well as an appreciation for differing family coping strategies. It is equally important to convince the school personnel that even a child with a serious illness continues to achieve and develop and may have years of valuable life ahead. Hope is essential in dealing with these students. Unlike denial, hope does not interfere with healthy adjustment and is entirely compatible with an acceptance of reality.

Van Eys states that when caregivers do not expect cure, they hamper development. Some may expect the child to die and, therefore, do not do what is demanded to help the child develop. This attitude, which Van Eys labels, "psychological euthanasia," may serve to protect caregivers, but is devastating to the child in the classroom (Van Eys, 1977). It is imperative, then, that teachers be helped to see the child with cancer as a living, growing, developing child valiantly trying to learn in spite of a difficult situation.

Specific Issues Relative to School

We have found that most children with cancer have difficulties in school for a variety of reasons. Some children, for example, have reading problems. Teachers who see the child as living despite the cancer refer for appropriate diagnostic evaluation and remediation. Teachers who see the child as dying do not refer, and the child goes from grade to grade carrying the burden, not only of illness, but also of a worsening reading difficulty. Attendance may be a problem because of clinic visits and occasional hospitalizations. Many teachers are very cooperative and flexible and allow the child to make up work. Others, especially at the secondary level, do not. The adolescent's need for privacy, coupled with a teacher's need for an excuse for absence, can often conflict, especially when an adequate communication system is not present in the school to inform all teachers, not only of the fact of the illness, but also of the consequences as they apply to school work.

A well-prepared teacher is a valuable link in the total care of the child. Prepared to deal with the family in crisis, as well as the child, teachers are in a position to communicate with parents in a way health care professionals might not be. For example, many children with cancer were diagnosed as toddlers and preschoolers. Entering into school is a significant step, not only for these children, but also for their parents. If the child is successful, the parents feel rewarded in their efforts to promote normal growth and development in spite of the illness. If the child has problems, parents too frequently link these problems to the cancer, and blame the cancer for noncancer related difficulties. A well-prepared teacher will point out to these parents that many children have difficulties at the beginning, not only a child with cancer. This support of the parents at a critical transition time by a competent teacher helps the child. In addition, teachers can help parents recognize developmental problems for what they are. The transition from elementary to junior high school is stressful for all students, not merely for the student with cancer.

School is particularly significant for the adolescent cancer patient. The diagnosis of the disease and its treatment can prevent or impede successful development of autonomy, acquisition of consistent body image and sex roles, establishment of peer relations, and the adoption of future-orientated social and intellectual preparation (Kellerman & Katz, 1977).

It is important, then, to allow the adolescent to maximize his or her own sense of control. School is one area where the adolescent cancer patient can exercise such control. It is essential that all the school personnel with whom the teenager interacts—teachers, counselors, administrators, school nurse—understand not only the fact of the illness, but its school-related consequences as they apply specifically to the adolescent.

In brief, school is an important part of the life of the child with cancer. A well-prepared teacher, one who is attempting to come to terms with her own philosophy of life, who understands the medical facts specific to her student, who sees the child as living, growing, and developing toward a very real future, and who understands the dynamics of the child's family, is in an excellent position to make school a positive, happy place for the child.

Children with cancer are living longer and attending school in the regular classroom. It is necessary to prepare school personnel at all levels to assume an active role in the total care of the child. This preparation goes far beyond the mere transmission of pertinent medical facts. It involves helping teachers, counselors, administrators, and school nurses to come to terms with their own philosophy of life and death, to understand the psychosocial implication of the illness for the child, and to appreciate the stress on the parents. It is essential to convince educators that the child with cancer is a living, growing person with a future. School personnel need to know that the members of the health care team are there to support them and are available to work through any difficulties the teacher, student, or parent may be experiencing.

Since children with cancer are living longer and seeking a normal life by attending school, communication with the school becomes not a luxury, but a vital and essential element in the total care of the child. Everyone involved benefits from expanded communication with the child's school: the child is happier in school; teachers are more comfortable in their role; the parents are content that the child is safe, productive, and functioning just like any other child his age; and the physician gets a more complete picture of the child. Teachers and other school personnel play a significant role in the life of the child with cancer. Given adequate preparation, information, and support, they are an essential and invaluable link in the total care of the child.

CONCLUSIONS

The health care setting for the child with cancer is three-fold: the hospital (with its out-patient clinics), the family, and the school. All three elements must be addressed if effective communication is to take place. To expect to communicate with a child about his or her diagnosis, treatment, and prognosis without taking into account the child's primary growth environments, is to fail to communicate with that child. What we have attempted to demonstrate in this chapter is the necessity for making parents and teachers an integral part of the total health care team. We have attempted to outline, in some detail, both theoretical and practical approaches to the issue of communication between health care professionals and the child with cancer. Hopefully, some of these thoughts and concerns will support others in their efforts at helping a child with cancer lead as full, happy, and normal a life as possible within the physical limits imposed by the illness. Children with cancer can lead fulfilled lives.

REFERENCES

Alby, N., and Alby, J. M. The doctor and the dying child. In E. J. Anthony and C. Koupernik (Eds.), *The Child in His Family,* Vol. 2: *The Impact of Disease and Death.* New York: John Wiley & Sons, Inc., 1973.

Aradine, C. R. Books for children about death. *Pediatrics,* 57, 372-377, 1976.

Axelrod, B. H. The chronic care specialist: "But who supports us?" In O. J. Z. Sahler (Ed.), *The Child and Death.* St. Louis: C. V. Mosby Co., 1978.

Binger, C. M., Ablin, A. R., Feuerstein, R. C. et al. Childhood leukemia; Emotional impact on patient and family. *New England Journal of Medicine,* 280, 414-418, 1969.

Bluebond-Langner, M. I know, do you?: Awareness and communication in terminally ill children. In B. Schoenberg, A. Carr, D. Peretz, and A. Kutscher (Eds.), *Anticipatory Grief.* New York: Columbia University Press, 1974.

Clapp, M. J. Psychosocial reactions of children with cancer. *Nursing Clinics of North America,* 11, 73-78, 1976.

Easson, W. M. *The Dying Child: The Management of the Child or Adolescent who is Dying.* Springfield: Charles C Thomas, Publisher, 1970.

Feifel, H. Death in contemporary America. In H. Feifel (Ed.), *New Meanings of Death.* New York: McGraw-Hill Book Co., 1977.

Futterman, E. J., and Hoffman, I. Crisis and adaptation in the families of fatally ill children. In E. J. Anthony and C. Koupernik (Eds.), *The Child in His Family: The Impact of Disease and Death,* Vol. 2. *The Yearbook of the International Association for Child Psychiatry and Allied Professions.* New York: John Wiley & Sons, Inc., 1973.

Glock, C. Y. *Religion and Society in Tension*. Chicago: Rand McNally & Co., 1965.
Grollman, E. A. (Ed.). *Explaining Death to Children*. Boston: Beacon Press, Inc., 1967.
Hansen, Y. *Development of the Concept of Death: Cognitive Aspects*. (Los Angeles: California School of Professional Psychology, 1972). Ann Arbor: University Microfilms, 1973. (73-19, 640).
Hofer, M. A., Wolff, C. T., Friedman, S. B., and Mason, J. W. A psychoendocrine study of bereavement, Part I: 17-Hydroxycorticosteroid excretion rates of parents following death of their children from leukemia. *Psychosomatic Medicine*, 34, 481-507, 1972.
Hostler, S. L. The development of the child's concept of death. In O. J. Z. Sahler (Ed.), *The Child and Death*. St. Louis: C. V. Mosty, Co., 1978.
Howarth, R. The psychiatric care of children with life-threatening illnesses. In L. Burton (Ed.), *Care of the Child Facing Death*. Boston: Routledge & Kegan Paul, Ltd., 1974.
Jackson, E. N. *Telling a Child about Death*. New York: Hawthorn Books, Inc., 1965.
Kantor, D., and Lehr, W. *Inside the Family*. San Francisco: Jossey-Bass, Publishers, 1975.
Kastenbaum, R. Death and development through the lifespan. In H. Feifel (Ed.), *New Meanings of Death*. New York: McGraw-Hill Book Co., 1977.
Kellerman, J., and Katz, E. R. The adolescent with cancer: Theoretical, clinical, and research issues. *Journal of Pediatric Psychology*, 2(3), 127, 1977.
Kellerman, J., Rigler, D., Siegel, S. E., and Katz, E. R. Disease-related communication and depression in pediatric cancer patients. *Journal of Pediatric Psychology*, 2(2), 52-53, 1977.
Koocher, G. P., and Sallan, S. E. Psychological issues in pediatric oncology. In P. R. Magrab (Ed.), *Psychological Management of Pediatric Problems*. (2 Vols.) Baltimore: University Park Press, 1978.
Lansky, S. B., Cairns, N. U., Hassanein, R., Wehr, J., and Lowman, J. R. Childhood cancer: Parental discord and divorce. *Pediatrics*, 62, 184-188, 1978.
Lansky, S. B., and Lowman, J. T. Childhood malignancy. *Journal of the Kansas Medical Society*, 75, 91-96, 1974.
Lazarus, R. S., and Launier, R. *Stress-related transactions between person and environment*. Unpublished manuscript, University of California, Berkeley, 1979.
Lecron, L. M. *Self-hypnotism: The Technique and Its use in Daily Living*. Englewood Cliffs, New Jersey: Prentice-Hall, 1964.
Lewis, J., Beavers, W., Gossett, J., and Phillips, V. *No Single Thread: Psychological Health in Family Systems*. New York: Brunner/Mazel, Inc., 1976.
Mussen, P. H., Conger, J. J., and Kagan, J. *Child Development and Personality*. 4th Ed. New York: Harper & Row Pubs., Inc., 1974.
Sahler, O. J. Z. Introduction. In O. J. Z. Sahler (Ed.), *The Child and Death*. St. Louis: C. V. Mosby, Co., 1978.
Schowalter, J. E. The reactions of caregivers dealing with fatally ill children and

their families. In O. J. Z. Sahler (Ed.), *The Child and Death*. St. Louis: C. V. Mosby, Co., 1978.

Selye, H. *Stress without Distress*. Philadelphia: Lippincott, 1974.

Selye, H. *The Stress of Life*. Rev. Ed. New York: NcGraw-Hill Book Co., 1976.

Sheposh, J. P., Spinetta, J. J., Chadwick, D. L., and Elliott, E. S. *Parental participation in decisions regarding extraordinary life-sustaining measures*. Unpublished manuscript, San Diego State University, 1978.

Spinetta, J. J. The dying child's awareness of death: A review. *Psychological Bulletin, 81*, 256-260, 1974.

Spinetta, J. J. Adjustment in children with cancer. *Journal of Pediatric Psychology, 2*(2), 49-51, 1977.

Spinetta, J. J. Communication patterns in families dealing with life-threatening illness. In O. J. Z. Sahler (Ed.), *The Child and Death*. St. Louis: C. V. Mosby, Co., 1978.

Spinetta, J. J. Disease-related communication: How to tell. In J. Kellerman (Ed.), *Psychological Aspects of Childhood Cancer*. Springfield, Illinois: Charles C Thomas, Publisher, 1979 (in press).

Spinetta, J. J., and Maloney, L. J. Death anxiety in the out-patient leukemic child. *Pediatrics, 56*, 1034-1037, 1975.

Spinetta, J. J., and Maloney, L. J. The child with cancer: Patterns of communication and denial. *Journal of Consulting and Clinical Psychology, 48*, 1540-1541, 1978.

Spinetta, J. J., Rigler, D., and Karon, M. Anxiety in the dying child. *Pediatrics, 52*, 841-845, 1973.

Spinetta, J. J., Rigler, D., and Karon, M. Personal space as a measure of the dying child's sense of isolation. *Journal of Consulting and Clinical Psychology, 42*, 751-756, 1974.

Spinetta, J. J., Spinetta, P. D., Kung, F., and Schwartz, D. B. *Emotional Aspects of Childhood Cancer and Leukemia: A Handbook for Parents*. San Diego: Leukemia Society of America, 1976.

Spinetta, J. J., Swarner, J., Kard, T., and Sheposh, J. P. *Effective parental coping following the death of a child from cancer*. Unpublished manuscript, San Diego State University, 1978.

Stehbens, J. A., and Lascari, A. D. Psychological follow-up of families with childhood leukemia. *Journal of Clinical Psychology, 30*, 394-396, 1974.

Toch, R. Too young to die. In B. Schoenberg, A. Carr, D. Peretz and A. Kutscher (Ed.), *Psychosocial Aspects of Terminal Care*. New York: Columbia University Press, 1972.

Townes, B., Wold, D., and Holmes, T. Parental adjustment to childhood leukemia. *Journal of Psychosomatic Research, 18*(1), 9-16, 1974.

Toynbee, A. Various ways in which human beings have sought to reconcile themselves to the fact of death. In E. S. Shneidman (Ed.), *Death: Current Perspectives*. Palo Alto: Mayfield Publishing Co., 1976.

Van Eys, J. What do we mean by "the truly cured child?" In J. van Eys (Ed.), *The*

Truly Cured Child: The New Challenge in Pediatric Cancer Care. Baltimore: University Park Press, 1977.

Viles, P. H. Reflections of a physician caregiver. In O. J. Z. Sahler (Ed.), *The Child and Death.* St. Louis: C. V. Mosby Co., 1978.

Waechter, E. H. Children's awareness of fatal illness. *American Journal of Nursing, 71,* 1168-1172, 1971.

Chapter 13

THE ROLE OF COMMUNICATIONS IN CHRONIC PAIN

Christine O. Mathews

Chronic pain patients present a complex and unique challenge to health professionals. The chronicity of pain presents additional problems beyond those faced by patients in acute crisis. Complexity is increased by the confusion stemming from usage of the word "pain." "Pain" refers to unpleasant physical sensations, but the experience of pain may vary greatly in intensity, quality, duration, and physical site. Furthermore, the experience of pain is subjective; the presence of pain is inferred on the basis of a varied group of behaviors that may be called "pain behavior." Pain behavior includes responses such as reflexive withdrawal or pulling one's hand away from heat as well as behaviors that are more individual and influenced by situational and cultural factors. Examples of this behavior include requesting medication, contacting a physician, resting, crying, and so forth. The focus in this chapter will be on the latter subgroup of pain behaviors, the meaning the pain may have for an individual, and how the individual may use pain and associated behaviors to influence and communicate with other people and to define his self-concept and social role. The emphasis will be on chronic pain patients rather than acute pain patients for several reasons. In the chronic patient, as opposed to the acute patient, pain and pain behavior assumes varied and complex meaning and function. Correspondingly, therapy of the chronic patient requires a rather different process with regard to the implicit or explicit treatment contract, the role of the patient in therapy, and in the roles of the health professionals.

At what point a patient becomes a chronic pain patient is certainly a subjective one. With respect to somatic etiology, a chronic, relatively benign process is implied rather than an acute time-limited or life-threatening process. Somatogenic as well as psychogenic pain may be found in a group of chronic pain patients. A distinction between the types of pain is both difficult to make and often arbitrary; more often they coexist. And, indeed, the experience of the pain is the same, whether psychogenic or somatogenic. Psychogenic pain refers both to conversion and psychophysiological reactions, e.g., headaches in absence of causative physical changes and tension headaches related to muscular contractions. Examples of chronic pain with physical origin include low back pain, peripheral neuropathies, arthritis, etc. However, even when the physical pathology can be identified, often little is available in the way of permanent treatment. In addition, the pain is often compounded by iatrogenic effects of the medical intervention. Thus the prospects for a definitive cure and relief for the chronic pain patient offer little room for optimism. A spiral of continued pain, accompanying fatigue and anxiety, and increasing salience of the pain as the patient focuses more and more of his attention on his symptoms are often the factors which lead to chronic sick role behavior and the person's increasing reference to the pain for his identity. His physician, diagnostic procedures, and medical interventions also become the focus of his attention. A cycle of searching for relief, somatic preoccupation, depression, helplessness, and passivity becomes entrenched.

Various models for understanding the pain and the psychological meaning it has for the patient have been proposed. Szasz (1957, 1959), for example, proposes a model which outlines three levels of the meaning of pain. In the first level, the pain is a symptom representing the anxiety and pain a person experiences whenever an important function, emotional or physical, is lost. On the second level, the patient uses pain as a means of communication or mode of interpersonal behavior with the primary goal of soliciting help. Szasz identifies the third level as symbolic in which the person uses the pain indirectly to manipulate other people and obtain other secondary gains. The distinction between the latter seems blurred as both represent pain used as a communication—a means of conveying some information to others or obtaining some response from them.

Another approach to understanding the meaning of pain and its function draws upon social role and social learning theories. An individual's self-concept and behavior in various situations can be understood in terms of different roles whose limits are defined by various cultural, situational, and individual factors. Common roles include those of the "husband," "wife," "son," "daughter," "student" as well as "patient" and "doctor." At various times an individual may function in various roles. For the chronic pain patient the role of patient or sick role often becomes the dominant one.

In our culture being "sick" entitles a person to special treatment. When ill, a person is excused from a variety of responsibilities including vocational, interpersonal, and emotional ones. Labeling one's self as sick communicates many different messages such as "I need extra attention" or "You can't expect as much from me." For example, when a person is ill, he is not expected to work, nor to care for his children in the same fashion. Responsibilities as husband or wife such as household chores and sex may be avoided. Beyond that, the patient typically benefits by receiving extra attention, nurturing care, narcotics, or often financial reward in terms of disability payments. By excusing the person from responsibilities and by giving him special treatment, others are also communicating messages such as "You have special needs; you cannot take care of yourself" and "Someone else must have responsibility for you." These communications confirm the patient's sick role identity and with the chronic patient make successful treatment of chronic pain very difficult.

Often individuals also use physical symptoms as a means of communicating psychological and emotional stress. The physical symptoms may be used as a substitute for emotional problems or a mechanism to avoid dealing with the problems directly.

The substitution may stem from an attitude that psychological problems are somehow not acceptable, whereas physical illness is. In some cases, people have not learned to identify feelings and emotions and the concept of emotional upset has, in a sense, never been learned. The person often lacks even the vocabulary to identify and express feelings. Instead the individual learns to use physical symptoms and illness as a means of avoiding conflicts yet communicating distress and influencing people.

Both Szasz (1968) and Berne (1964) elaborate the use of pain in interpersonal communications by describing specific types of sick role behavior or "games." For example, Szasz uses the term "painmenship" to describe a communication between pain patients and physicians. The physician, in the "doctor role," is invested in maintaining that identity by diagnosing the illness or pain and by treating the illness and alleviating the pain. The patient, too, is invested in his "sick role," but the degree of investment and its impact on his treatment procedure is not often recognized. In fact, the patient often may be as invested in maintaining his role as is the physician. Correspondingly, Szasz argues that it is no more likely that the patient would give up his identity than it would be for the physician to change his. As a consequence, an ultimately self-defeating pattern evolves. The patient pursues medical intervention to confirm his role as a patient, while at the same time protesting that he wants relief. The physician, confirming his role as doctor, responds with a series of futile medical interventions with increasing frustration for both patient and doctor. The pattern can be difficult to detect, however, as it is difficult to identify when the patient is using his pain in this fashion for psychological gain and when he is not.

Berne, in *Games People Play* (1964), describes various games that relate to the types of interactions many pain patients use. Examples include "Wooden Leg" or "What do you expect of a man with a wooden leg" and "Veteran" or "I got my rights." Sternbach (1974) elaborates on Berne's thesis and illustrates various "pain games," most of which would be readily recognizable by health professionals. He describes the basic pain game with the following transactions:

Pain patient: I hurt, please fix me. (But you can't.)
Doctor: I'll fix you.

Medical intervention fails; more interventions or a referral is made with continuing failure.

Pain patient (righteous indignation): Another incompetent quack.
Doctor (defensively): Another crock.

Sternbach describes the "home tyrant" as the individual who gets his way by using his pain as a weapon.

> Pain patient: It's not that I don't want to (put out the trash, have sex, go to work) I can't.
> Spouse: That's all right, dear. I understand.

"Somatizer" represents the patient who experiences physical instead of emotional pain and insists that everything in his life is "wonderful."

> Doctor: I imagine this has been quite a strain not only on you, but on your wife too, and you've had to make some adjustments.
> Pain patient: We've taken it all in stride, no problems. Of course I'm still trying to get relief; this pain never lets up.
> Doctor: Have you noticed that sometimes the pain seems worse when you're worried about things or you get upset?
> Pain patient: No, I can't say I have. I don't worry about anything. The only thing that bothers me is this pain. Everything would be fine if only this pain (headache, backache) would go away.

The basic factors in all the games, however, are the same. A person has experienced chronic pain, psychogenic or somatogenic, and evolves an identity as a chronic patient and suffering person. Subsequently, as the scope of his life narrows his goal becomes maintenance and confirmation of his identity. What differs among these individuals is the goal or type of secondary gain they are receiving that may include avoiding responsibility, manipulating other people, satisfying dependency needs, obtaining narcotics, receiving financial remuneration in the form of disability benefits, litigating suits, avoiding intimacy with others, avoiding emotional problems, and so forth.

The problem for the health professional, thus, becomes one of determining the meaning the pain has for the individual, his degree of investment in sick-role behaviors, the importance of the secondary gain; and how he uses his pain and associated symptoms to communicate with other people. The diagnosis of psychogenic versus somatogenic pain is often quite difficult to make, particularly as often they coexist. Various people, e.g., Sternbach, 1968; Szasz, 1957; Mersky & Spear, 1967, have argued that rather than classifying a pain as physical or emotional in origin, it is more useful to describe the problem in both psychological and physical terms and then pursue both psychological and medical treatment at the same time. Both psychological and physiological diagnostic procedures would thus be implemented simultaneously so as not to deny the person with organic etiology the opportunity to have the psychological factors assessed and treated and as not to imply inadvertently that the person without identifiable organic etiology is somehow not really sick or not really in pain. The reality, however, of many medical settings does not permit this parallel approach. Cultural attitudes and medical biases tend to support an "either-or" dichotomy along with the accompanying tendency to dismiss the person without obvious organic etiology as a "crock," crazy, or malingering. Furthermore, the confusion about psychogenic versus somatogenic pain is compounded by the iatrogenic effects of medical treatment of what might originally have been essentially a psychological problem.

To provide an adequate evaluation, a thorough physical assessment is required both to insure that appropriate medical intervention is provided and to reassure the patient that physical etiology has been thoroughly investigated. Chronic sick role patients may be more likely to accept involvement of a psychological process once they are satisfied that the medical review has been complete. Psychological assessment requires a thorough interview, with questions concerning current emotional stresses as well as stresses that may have coincided with the onset of the symptoms. Potential reinforcers or secondary gain for sick role behavior must be thoroughly examined; some examples of common secondary gains have been mentioned.

Often the simple question, "What would you do if you were well; how would things be different?" provides useful information. Essentially the goal is to determine what meaning the patient's pain and symptoms have for him, to what extent he identifies himself in terms of a sick role, and how he uses his pain to communicate and to influence other people. For example, the degree of involvement in other activities and interests may reflect his capacity to see himself in roles other than that of a patient. Do complaints about physical pain seem to be a substitute for expression of some emotional distress? Is the pain used to influence other people rather than direct communications about needs and feelings?

Factors that might predispose a person to psychogenic pain need to be evaluated, including the attitudes the person has learned concerning physical illness and emotional and behavioral disturbances along with the attitudes his family has about these disorders. Prior experience with the symptoms, perhaps through other family members having had the same symptoms, prior illness or injury, or association with the medical field may have provided the patient with the opportunity to learn the specific symptoms. Often psychological testing, such as the CPI-MMPI, is useful to help answer some of these questions and complete the psychological assessment.

In addition, obtaining an estimate of the degree of pain is important. Sometimes this information is obtained by asking the patient such questions as "On a scale of one to ten, what is your pain level now?; "What is the usual level of pain?"; "What do you do if the pain reaches an eight or nine level; a two or three level?" and so forth. It should be remembered, however, that such self-report measures are often inaccurate. A variety of experimental pain measures can be used to introduce physical pain to which the patient can compare his clinical pain, e.g., Woodforde & Merskey, 1972. Sternbach (1974) describes in more detail a submaximum effort tourniquet technique which he recommends that provides more reliable objective estimates.

Although the diagnostic process is an ongoing process, after the initial evaluation the health professional should carefully discuss with the patient treatment goals and procedures. Essentially the goal of treatment is to reduce the pain behavior and to increase goal-directed, healthy activities that are incompatible with pain; specific goals are negotiated with the individual. The importance of clarity of communication in this discussion cannot be over-emphasized. Unfortunately, in most health care settings, the treatment contract and the understanding and expectations of the patient and his physician remain covert. With most patients, making the treatment contract explicit facilitates therapy. With chronic pain patients, explicit discussion of expectations is critical as these patients have often been seen by many physicians and have often been disappointed. Along with their investment in maintaining their sick role identity, they may expect failure, thus adding a further obstacle to their progress. Another potential impediment is the accumulation of anger, following these disappointments, of which the patient may or may not be aware but which he probably has difficulty expressing directly. Unless these feelings are clarified and the patient encouraged to express them directly, additional passive-aggressive, passive-dependent behaviors may complicate the course of therapy.

Assumptions about goals and expectations should not be taken for granted. Even apparently basic issues should be discussed including such questions as does the patient want to reduce his pain and will the patient work at his therapy. A particular problem is that the patient typically expects to give up responsibility for his treatment and to give that responsibility to the health professionals. This expectation has been reinforced by cultural attitudes and the medical profession. Even the word "patient" itself connotes the idea that the ill individual places himself in the hands of the physician, "patiently" awaiting a cure. Successful therapy, however, requires that the patient assume responsibility for his treatment and takes a very active role in the treatment process both in terms of determining goals and implementing procedures. This transition from passivity to active involvement may be difficult to make as the former expectation may be deeply entrenched. Nevertheless, the importance of this transition for successful therapy is critical.

Reviewing the different treatment procedures with their specific goals enables the patient to have a clear understanding of the processes and facilitates active cooperation. Among the procedures typically employed with chronic pain patients are operant conditioning techniques, described elsewhere in detail, e.g. Fordyce et al., 1968, 1973, which emphasize removing the variables that reward pain behavior, such as attention, sympathy, medication, and rest and instead use comparable reinforcers to reward pain-incompatible activities. For example, health care staff attempt to ignore complaints of pain and to reward activity, such as increasing time out of bed, with attention or conversation.

Other dimensions of the therapy, which are equally important, relate more directly to problems of communication. Essential to the treatment is the patient learning to communicate to others directly, both professional staff and family and friends, rather than through physical complaints. For example, rather than saying "I hurt, I need some medication," he might learn instead to say, more accurately, "I'm sad, please talk to me" or "I don't like what you're doing; could you please stop." Group therapy and family therapy is often very helpful in clarifying how the patient uses his pain to communicate to and manipulate other people. Assertiveness training, discussed in another chapter, provides an excellent opportunity for direct relearning of communication skills. The goals are to help the patient learn to identify feelings, rights, and responsibilities and express them directly while respecting the rights of other people. Additional benefits of assertiveness training are improved self-concept and a sense of having increased control over one's life, factors which also relate to the patient's willingness to assume an involved, responsible role in his therapy.

Including the physician or surgeon at occasional group meetings is also helpful. These interactions provide an opportunity for the patients to learn how to communicate more directly with these health professionals. Data indicating or contraindicating medical intervention, both physical and emotional, along with probabilities of success and failure, can be discussed openly. Medical procedures can come to be understood more as problem solving which depends on the patient's involvement and cooperation efforts rather than magical cures.

Biofeedback training is another very useful treatment modality, particularly with patients whose pain relates to a psychophysiological process or in whom tension and anxiety lowers their threshold of pain. Biofeedback training helps the patient recognize the association between tension and pain and then learn how to reduce the tension and thus alleviate the pain. With different psychophysiologic reactions, one type of biofeedback information may be more useful than another, e.g., hand temperature and vascular headaches. Specific methods and applications of biofeedback training have been discussed extensively elsewhere, e.g., Brown, 1976; Gaarder & Montgomery, 1977. A point worth emphasizing, however, is that biofeedback training does not act upon the patient but merely facilitates his learning a skill that requires frequent practice and individual effort but that can provide considerable control over physiological processes.

The two following case examples describe two patients whose

primary complaints were chronic pain, both psychogenic and somatogenic. They were treated primarily as inpatients on a behaviorally-oriented milieu unit in a respected diagnostic clinic, a tertiary care hospital. Available treatment components included traditional group therapy, assertiveness training groups, biofeedback, role-playing, intensive individual therapy, family therapy, and recreation and art therapy. Patients, not exclusively pain patients, with various psychophysiological and conversion reactions were treated on this service as well as patients whose primary problems were emotional and behavioral.

Case Example, Mrs. J. S.

When J. first contacted the clinic, she was twenty-six years old, married, with three children. Her presenting complaints were severe headaches that "never go away" and have lasted for three-and-a-half years. She described being in almost constant state of nausea with vomiting occurring when the pain became unbearable. Headaches were accompanied by neck, shoulder, and facial soreness and tenderness, along with other sore and tender areas over the rest of her body. Occasionally, she also experienced severe weakness in limbs and temporary blindness. She recognized that tension and anxiety may have been a factor in her headaches but had been treated with antidepressant and pain medication with no results. Prior neurological studies were essentially normal, as was the neurological evaluation she received at the clinic. The neurology service then referred the patient to psychology to be evaluated for biofeedback training for treatment of her headaches. During the psychology interview, it became apparent that, in addition to having headaches, the patient was quite depressed, able to function only with considerable difficulty, and was actively considering suicide. Stresses included marital problems (her current marriage was her third marriage), traumatic early background, and an overinvolved, manipulative family. Psychological testing, CPI-MMPI, pointed mainly to an egocentric, alienated, passive-aggressive, passive-dependent, manipulative character disorder. Her usual means of coping apparently were not working for her, a fact reflected in much diffuse upset and schizoid qualities in the testing. Hospitalization on the psychology service on the milieu unit was recommended. The patient was quite amenable to this recommendation although her husband was rather skeptical. Her husband conveyed an attitude of general disgust with the patient and pessimism for her capacity for change. Similarly, he was not interested in marital therapy but expressed the feeling that before they worked on the marriage his wife would have to deal with her own personality problems.

The pain J. was experiencing in her headaches was, in a sense, symbolic of her low self-esteem and her concept of herself as a long-suffering person. Indeed, there seemed to be some truth to this claim as the patient described a very chaotic and traumatic family background, with emotionally disturbed parents, that was rife with faulty communication patterns and many mixed messages. J. attributed some of her parents' disturbed behavior to their having been victims of a concentration camp in the Far East. Understanding their problems did not mitigate the destructive family atmosphere. Although her father violently abused her mother and brothers, his treatment of J. was relatively good, provided she stayed within certain well-defined limits—i.e. remained a conventional, sweet, acquiescent girl/doll. Her mother, however, displaced much of her anger on J. While her father rewarded her for seductive, manipulative behavior her mother accused her, without foundation, of sexual promiscuity. Eventually J. married at sixteen to escape the home situation. The chaos culminated in a brother killing her father in self-defense. Generally maladaptive relationships continued among remaining family members with much double-bind manipulative communications.

As a consequence, J. emerged with generally low self-esteem, extreme difficulty in communicating directly with anyone, and a reliance on passive-aggressive and manipulative behavior to influence other people.

She used her headaches in a similar fashion—to manipulate her children and husband. Her children learned to be quiet and to take care of themselves fairly well despite their ages (nine, seven, and six) and, thus, reinforced her headaches. With respect to her husband, J. seemed to employ the headaches as a form of rather masochistic retaliation to his rather distant, distrustful, critical attitude toward her. With a headache, she would assume an abject, suffering attitude, withdraw, and stop household-related tasks; all of which irritated her husband enormously. Although she recognized the marital problems, the headaches provided her with an excuse for not dealing with them directly. In addition, the headaches provided an excuse for not seeking employment or continuing education. Despite the fact that she was capable, her reluctance seemed to relate more to a lack of self-confidence than a dislike of work itself, although not being able to work provided her with an additional reason for not being able to leave her husband. Much of her identity was invested in being sick. Partially due to her husband's disapproval, her subservience and lack of self-confidence, she had stopped working, stopped seeing her friends, and gradually reduced the scope of her other activities and interests. Since her marriage, her involvement as a mother with her children was quite important and her sick role had not continued so long as to be completely entrenched.

Focus of therapy on the milieu unit, in which the patient participated actively, was on issues of self-esteem and learning to communicate her feelings directly, rather than relying on passive-aggressive and passive-dependent modes of interaction. With continued biofeedback training, J.

learned to achieve considerable muscular control with significant relaxation; yet, nevertheless, complained of headaches even in biofeedback sessions, which suggested a conversion component to her headaches, as well as the psychophysiologic dimension. J. did feel, however, that at times she could use the skill she had learned in biofeedback training to abort headaches. At the time of discharge, the patient's headaches as well as her depression were considerably alleviated.

Continuing problems included difficulty with communicating directly and her seductive, manipulative behaviors with men. For example, she continued to have a great deal of difficulty expressing any anger or displeasure toward her husband for fear of further jeopardizing the marriage. Her relationships with male staff and male patients tended to be flirtatious and seductive. Occasionally, her statement to staff about her feelings in a particular situation would be contradictory. After discharge, follow-up with individual therapy was recommended although, unfortunately, frequent contacts were made difficult by the distance between J.'s home and the hospital.

Approximately two-and-a-half months later, J. requested readmission to the milieu unit with the presenting complaints of depression and several somatic complaints, in particular rather diffuse bruising. Although J. denied any physical trauma, the question of the bruising being self-inflicted was considered a possibility. The conclusion of the consultation with the medical service was that the bruises probably were iatrogenic, a consequence of medication with meprobamate. J. continued working during hospitalization on many of the same issues as during the previous hospitalization. Her husband believed she was overly dependent on the unit and was using hospitalization as an escape; he threatened a divorce if she stayed. J.'s decision to continue the hospitalization reflected greater self-confidence in her ability to cope, alone if need be. Correspondingly, she was able to be more assertive with her husband, who respected her assertiveness. She was also more assertive with her family and was able to withdraw from the pathological relationships. A significant portion of her husband's dissatisfaction related to her overinvolvement and subservience to her family as well as her abject passive-dependent behavior toward him. To the extent that she was more assertive and communicated feelings directly, the marital relationship improved.

Furthermore, she investigated various continuing education and employment opportunities and accepted an office managerial position that entailed significant responsibility and provided her with satisfaction. She also resumed other interests and activities beyond the limits of her house and husband, thus providing herself with a variety of options beyond a sick role. Although she still retained many of her former maladaptive means of coping, she made an important beginning in learning other modes of coping; certainly she had moved beyond her identity as a pain patient and a reliance upon her pain for communication.

Case Example, Mrs. D. K.

When psychological consultation was first requested, D. K. was a forty-year-old married woman who had been separated from her husband for approximately seven years. Previously she had been employed as an R.N., although she had been receiving disability payment for approximately the last five years. At the time of the consultation, she was living with her mother, an aunt, and a female friend of the family, who was approximately D's age. The patient had a fourteen-year history of upper gastrointestinal pain with associated nausea and other general somatic complaints, considered by the medical services to have a mixed conversion/psychophysiologic component. She had been a patient at the hospital for about ten years with multiple hospitalization on various services in which she received multiple surgeries and numerous nerve blocks. The somatogenic and psychogenic dimensions of the symptoms were impossible to sort out. In addition, the confusion was certainly compounded by the iatrogenic effects of previous medical intervention. The original surgery involved the removal of a portion of her stomach for treatment of ulcers. Although to some degree her multiple complaints, including many pain complaints and a wide variety of other symptoms from dizzyness, weakness, fatigue, to loss of appetite, may have been related to somatic etiology, certainly there was strong evidence of psychological contribution.

Psychological testing, CPI-MMPI, suggested a psychophysiologic basis for symptoms. The initial interview also revealed sufficient information to support a psychogenic component in her symptoms. Some secondary gain for a sick role was evident. For example, the patient admitted to a past history of alcohol abuse; review of medical records raised the question of narcotic dependency and certainly pointed to a general pattern of medication abuse. Relations with family members also appeared to be strained and a source of emotional stress. The patient, however, was quite reluctant to accept the idea that there might be a connection between psychological and emotional factors and her physical symptoms despite the fact that she was reassured that there was no intent to imply that her pain and other symptoms were not real. After the lapse of several months and an additional hospitalization, she agreed to be admitted to the milieu unit on the psychology service. She continued to be quite reluctant to consider emotional involvement in her problems and declined to participate in many of the milieu programs. Most of her therapy involved intensive, individual psychotherapy. Through the course of this therapy, considerable interpersonal and psychological problems emerged that illustrated how central her pain and physical symptoms were in her interpersonal relationships. Her identity was almost exclusively one of a sick, suffering person; she was thoroughly invested in a sick role. She had virtually no resources, no interests, or friends beyond the family limits. The course of her medical history had reinforced this sick-role identity. Her communications with physicians followed a particular pattern that was difficult to identify and easy to become involved with unwittingly. D. would typically exhibit some symptomatic relief following medical intervention, enough to encourage and engage continued medical efforts, yet the symptoms would invariably recur.

Despite her tendency to describe her relationships with her family as quite positive, in fact, her family, particularly her mother, was extremely domineering, manipulative, and guilt-provoking. The mother also used physical symptoms to manipulate and provoke guilt in D. D.'s only escape from the family tyranny was through physical illness. When she was sick, the family would indulge her and permit her to retire to her room. Otherwise she was not permitted to withdraw from the family where the general level of interactions was chaotic. With the exception of D., all the women were large people whose normal conversation consisted of everyone shouting at the same time; a pattern they demonstrated dramatically in a family therapy appointment. Much of the communication placed D. squarely in double-bind situations. For example, her mother would complain of chest pains, refuse to consult a physician, yet imply that D., as a nurse, should take care of her. She would also complain about housework, yet become angry if D. did anything to help. Examples of this type of communication were endless. Unfortunately, as the family lived a considerable distance from the hospital, regular family therapy was not feasible. There were few local resources as the home area was rather isolated.

Past history revealed that the patient had a rather isolated, schizoid childhood; currently her personality integration was borderline on the basis of the psychological assessment that was extended to include Rorschach and TAT testing. D.'s previous association with the medical profession as a nurse, history of family illnesses, and her own prior illnesses gave her a wide range of experience for learning many physical illnesses and pain behavior.

The nature of her relationship with her husband and her reasons for leaving the marriage, yet never divorcing him, were never entirely clear. Presumably they could not agree on whether to live in Ohio, where she was residing, or in North Carolina, where he had been living. As D. described the disagreement, he felt the weather was too cold in Ohio, and she said there were too many snakes in North Carolina! In fact, the marital problems appeared to be related to her ambivalence about sexual relationships. She had had in the past some homosexual experiences, as well, including a relationship with the female friend of the family who was living at the home. Although, at present, the relationship was presumable nonsexual, she experienced considerable guilt and conflict over her previous homosexual relationships and considerable immediate pressure from the friend who was quite possessive and domineering. D. felt herself to be incapable of relating to her family in any other role except as an invalid and was incapable of considering alternative means of dealing with her family or living outside the family situation.

Two subsequent admissions followed on the milieu unit again for depression and anxiety, as well as abdominal pain, nausea, and vomiting. On outpatient appointments, D. would arrive in a wheelchair. Her speech would be quite slurred and often unintelligible, but she could express desperate feelings of depression and helplessness. Upon arrival on the unit, she would immediately regain her strength, demonstrating an ability to walk and talk without any particular problems. Yet once in the unit, she would be reluctant to participate in milieu activities although she gradually acknowledged the relationship between her emotional and physical problems. Her third admission was allowed only with strict contingencies that she participate actively in the milieu and eliminate any use of narcotics. At this point, she did make gains in terms of participating in more ward activities, recognizing psychological problems, and learning to associate definite correlations between gastric and emotional upsets with some diminution of somatic complaints. She also made some progress in terms of working through her feelings about men and guilt about her sexuality. However, the course of therapy was disrupted by a change in hospital policies, prohibiting involvement of the psychology service with inpatients. Previously, she had been working primarily with the psychology service in the hospital. However, change in hospital policy required psychiatric services to be primary on in-hospital programs. Having developed a strong relationship with her original therapist and having begun to make some progress, she refused transfer to the psychiatric service and was discharged.

Again, due to the distance to her home, intensive outpatient psychotherapy was not feasible. Upon discharge, she returned home to essentially the same pathological situation and accompanying depression, sick-role behaviors, and pain patient identity.

She was again hospitalized on a medical service briefly and had a follow-up medical and psychological outpatient visit. In a phone contact with the psychology service, D. claimed that she had visited a local clinic and had been diagnosed as having a terminal liver disease with a six-to-eight month life expectancy. In the follow-up medical appointment noted, there was no definitive resolution to this question. An additional appointment was scheduled which the patient did not keep. There was no further contact with D. A follow-up phone call two years later indicated that the patient had died approximately one month after her last appointment. Accurate information was not available from her family to determine the cause of death.

D.'s situation reflects the close relationship of psychogenic, somatogenic, and iatrogenic pain as well as problems attendant to cultural biases toward mind-body dualism. Certainly psychological factors were crucial. With her marked tendency to somaticize, she used her pain as a symbolic communication of her emotional unhappiness. Despite the fact that her sick role was not working well for her, which she recognized, she saw no feasible alternative roles for coping. Her real physical limitations and her borderline level of personality adjustment did make her problems more difficult to resolve satisfactorily. Her investment in maintaining a sick role was almost desperate; her pain and other symptoms seemed to be the sole mode by which she could communicate to, and influence, family. They were the primary means of communication with others as well. She did make progress, albeit slowly, in decreasing her somaticization, communicating more directly, and even beginning to admit that alternatives might exist. Unfortunately, whether or not that progress would have continued is unknown.

Both D. and J. illustrate, however, how critically communication processes affect the experience of pain; the development of chronic pain behavior and sick role identities; and the function of pain on communication as a symbol of unhappiness and as a means of expressing needs and influencing people. Furthermore, they illustrate how altering communication patterns may be fundamental in the treatment of chronic pain. Learning to identify feelings and needs; learning to express needs directly; learning alternative methods of coping; and learning more alternative, adaptive behaviors to obtain the reinforcers that pain behavior previously obtained are often the most direct, most effective ways the health professional can help the chronic pain patient live a fuller, less painful life.

REFERENCES

Brown, B. *Stress and the Art of Biofeedback.* New York: Harper & Row, Pubs. Inc., 1976.

Fordyce, W. E., Fowler, R. S., Lehmann, J. F., and DeLatuer, B. J. Some implications of learning in problems of chronic pain. *Journal of Chronic Diseases, 21,* 79-190, 1958.

Fordyce, W. E., Fowler, R. S., Lehmann, J. F., Delatuer, B. J., Sand, P. L., and Trieschmann, R. B. Operant conditioning in the treatment of chronic pain. *Archives of Physical Medicine and Rehabilitation, 54,* 399-408, 1973.

Gaarder, K., and Montgomery, P. *Clinical Biofeedback: A Procedure Manual.* Baltimore: Williams & Wilkins Co., 1977.

Merskey, H., and Spear, F. G. *Pain: Psychological and Psychiatric Aspects.* London: Bailliere, Tindall and Cussell, 1967.

Soulairac, A., Cahn, J., and Carpenter, J. (Eds.). *Pain.* New York: Academic Press, Inc., 1968.

Sternbach, R. A. *Pain: A Psychophysiological Analysis*. New York: Academic Press, Inc., 1968.

Sternbach, R. A. *Pain Patients: Traits and Treatment*. New York: Academic Press, Inc., 1974.

Szasz, T. S. *Pain and Pleasure: A Study of Bodily Feelings*. New York: Basic Books, Inc., 1957.

Szasz, T. S. Language and pain. In S. Arieti (Ed.), *American Handbook of Psychiatry*, Vol. 1. New York: Basic Books, Inc., 1959.

Woodforde, J. M., and Mersky, H. Some relationships between subjective measures of pain. *Journal of Psychosomatic Research, 16*, 173-178, 1972.

Ziegler, F. J., Imboden, J. B., and Rodgers, D. A. Contemporary conversion reactions. *Journal of the American Medical Association, 188*, 307-311, 1963.

SECTION IV

In this final section, the focus shifts from theoretical and experiential aspects of communication to the problems of conducting empirical research on communication in health care settings. Attempts to quantify naturally-occurring aspects of communication or to measure the effects of communication training programs for health care professionals demonstrate the multiple problems faced by the researcher working in a health care setting. It is through controlled research that an empirical base will be established which will help improve communication patterns.

Chapter 14

SPINAL CORD INJURED PATIENTS' PERCEPTIONS OF WARD ATMOSPHERE FOLLOWING ASSERTIVENESS TRAINING OF NURSING STAFF

LaFaye C. Sutkin

The purpose of the present study was to determine whether assertiveness training of ward nursing staff would improve the spinal cord injured patient's perception of ward climate.

Ward climate refers to the psychosocial environment of a ward as distinct from physical facilities. It includes the human elements of a medical ward, such as warmth, understanding, helpfulness, encouragement, etc, (Jackson, 1969; Moos, 1968; Klagsburn, 1977; Moos, 1970). For several years the general psychosocial environment has been a subject of increasing concern on psychiatric wards (Moos, 1967, 1975; Hall, 1977; Jackson, 1969; Cohen & Struening, 1965). More recently, that concern has extended to medical-surgical units such as cancer units (Klagsburn, 1977), renal dialysis units, and intensive care units (Hay & Oken, 1972; Moos, 1976). Initially, investigators made only descriptive statements suggesting the importance of ward social structure in facilitating or hindering treatment goals. Subsequent to these efforts, attempts were made to measure various aspects of the treatment environment (Moos, 1968; Hall, 1977; Jackson, 1969). Moos and Houts (1973) developed a Ward Atmosphere Scale which assesses a ward's psychosocial treatment environment as perceived by both patients and staff, and Jackson (1969) provided a Characteristics of Treatment Environments Scale which described the environment of patients in a mental hospital. The perceived ward climate has been shown to correlate with some objective features of a ward, such as size and staffing (Moos, 1972). Most importantly, differences in ward rating scales have been demonstrated to be related to rates of discharge, community stays, readmission rates, and rehabilitation (Moos, 1970; Pierce, Trickett, & Moos, 1972; Linn, 1970). In general, it appears that a favorable ward atmosphere is associated with positive outcomes on psychiatric wards. In the course of investigations on psychiatric wards, certain factors or dimensions have emerged that appear to underlie favorable perceptions of ward climate. Moos has labeled dimensions associated with favorable ward climates as follows: (a) relationship, which includes support and spontaneity; (b) personal development, which includes autonomy, practical orientation, and personal problem orientation; and, finally, (c) system maintenance, which includes control, clarity, and structure (Moos, 1969).

Many of the interpersonal characteristics that underlie Moos' dimensions of a ward climate are similar to characteristics that have been demonstrated to alter as a result of assertiveness training (Eisler, Herson, Miller & Blanchard, 1973; Lange & Jakubowski, 1976; Rich & Schroeder, 1976). With regard to the relationship dimension, support would seem to involve increasing positive messages and decreasing negative messages. The spontaneity element of a relationship would seem to increase as a function of improved skill at "small talk" and increased "feeling talk," which have frequently been the focus of outcome studies in assertiveness (Zeichner, Wright, & Herman, 1977; Tigerman & Kassinove, 1977; Rich & Schroeder, 1976; Heimberg, Montgomery & Heimberg, 1977). With respect to the second major dimension, personal development, the characteristics of autonomy, practical orientation, and personal problem orientation, which make up the personal development dimension, should improve with improved skill in problem-solving and reduced anxiety in self-expression. Problem-solving has been shown to be more effective following assertiveness training (Corby, 1975; Wolpe, 1958; Scherer & Freedberg, 1976). And, reduced anxiety in self-expression is a relatively consistent finding in assertiveness training research (Rich & Schroeder, 1976; Tigerman & Kassinove, 1977). Finally, as regards the system maintenance dimension, control, clarity, and structure would be expected to ensue from improvement in communication skills, improved problem-solving capacity, and decreased anxiety in self-expression (Lange & Jakubowski, 1976; Rimm & Masters, 1975). In fact, research on alcoholic and psychiatric inpatient wards, as well as marital therapy research have shown assertiveness training to increase control and structure (Scherer & Freedberg, 1977; Lazarus & Serber, 1968, Witkin, 1976; Rich & Schroeder, 1976; Sarason, 1968). In general, measures of interpersonal relationships have been the focus of a number of investigations into the outcome of assertiveness training (Hersen, Eisler, Miller, Johnson, & Pinkston, 1974). In addition, individuals having undergone assertiveness training have increased their capacity to assume control and provide consistent and clear leadership (Flowers & Booraem, 1975; Heimberg, Montgomery & Heimberg, 1977; Carlson, 1976). In summary, assertiveness training leads to changes in relationship, personal development, and system maintenance and these dimensions appear related to perceived ward environment.

As yet, no single procedure for assertiveness training has been agreed upon (Flowers & Booraem, 1976; Rich & Schroeder, 1975; Heimberg, Montgomery & Heimberg, 1977). In many instances, single techniques such as viewing or visualizing assertive responses or practicing assertive responses are employed to alter one or two observable behaviors, such as making or refusing requests (Nietzel, Martorano & Meinick, 1977; Rosenthal & Reese, 1976; Janda & Rimm, 1977). Often, however, the problems are broader and more general than making or refusing requests, as is the case in marital conflicts or in patient groups where communications may be hampered by too many negative statements, too few positive statements, indirect requests, unwarranted assumptions or a failure to distinguish between aggression, assertion, and nonassertion (Witkin, 1976; Lange & Jakubowski, 1976; Tigerman & Massinove, 1977). Also, it is often the case that individuals such as shy women possess the desired skills for behaving assertively but are blocked in doing so by beliefs and attitudes which may be seen as irrational when they are discussed and examined (Lange & Jakubowski, 1976; Wolpe & Lazarus, 1966; Janda & Rimm, 1977; Ellis, 1975). When more extensive behavior change is sought or where beliefs or attitudes block performance, training usually consists of a combination of techniques such as modeling and role-playing with feedback provided by group members and trainers along with lectures and discussions (Heimberg, Montgomery, & Heimberg, 1977; Lange & Jakubowski, 1976; Alberti & Emmons, 1974; Rimm & Masters, 1974). The combination of a number of behavioral assertiveness training techniques with discussion of attitudes and lectures on basic rights is commonly called a cognitive-behavioral approach to assertiveness (Lange & Jakubowski, 1976).

An approach to assertiveness that combines role-playing, modeling, and practice, and lectures would appear most adaptable to the task of producing the variety of changes in interpersonal interactions including increases in positive messages and decreases in negative messages; greater spontaneity; more autonomy; improved practical and personal problem orientation; and greater control, structure, and clarity which Moos has suggested may underlie a favorable ward atmosphere (Moos, 1973). Lange & Jakubowski (1976) offer the most precise specifications of a cognitive-behavioral approach which combines assertiveness training techniques with discussions and lectures. According to Lange and Jakubowski, assertiveness training includes four basic procedures. The first procedure involves teaching people the difference between assertion and aggression and between nonassertion and politeness. For example, on a hospital ward, nursing staff might be asked to discriminate between an aggressive reply such as, "You have some nerve asking me to get you water now. Can't you see I'm busy? I'll get your water when I'm free." Or, nurses may be instructed in the difference between nonassertive behavior such as remaining silent when a patient is creating a disturbance and a polite request such as, "I understand that hospitals are boring places and that you've been here a long time, Mr._____, but your stereo is disturbing other patients and I'm going to have to ask you to lower the volume." A second goal of assertiveness training is helping people to identify and accept their own personal rights as well as the rights of others. In particular, the attention given to the rights of others would have relevance for the hospital setting. In a hospital, the relationship between nurses and patients is not equal in the way that marriage, dating, or social relationships might be. Nurses contract to provide care for and serve the needs of patients; whereas, patients are not required to meet the interpersonal needs of their nurses. On the other hand, nurses do possess rights that are occasionally ignored, such as the authority to make and enforce rules and the right to object to verbal or physical abuse. The third procedure described by Lange and Jakubowski is that of reducing cognitive and affective obstacles to acting assertively. Members of a nursing staff are likely to have an extensive repertoire of appropriate social skills but may be blocked in their performance by certain beliefs and attitudes (Ellis, 1975). For example, most nurses probably effectively handle sexual overtures outside of the hospital; however, a belief that she is there to serve the patient and that the patient is always right may interfere with an appropriate reaction in the hospital. Also, it is likely that nurses are able to refuse a request but find refusing a patient difficult, even when appropriate, because of the belief that the patient's hardships entitle him to have anything he wishes. Nurses who are capable of reciprocal interactions socially may patronize patients if they hold the attitude that illness causes individuals to become childlike. Often nurses are abrupt when issuing orders to a patient because they believe that authority may only be established by someone who sounds harsh. A discussion concerning the peculiar difficulties of certain types of patients and nurse-patient relationships would help to identify the attitudes and beliefs held by nurses and would offer an opportunity to repudiate irrational tenets. Finally, developing assertive skills such as increasing positive messages, "small talk," "feeling talk," and problem-solving skills and decreasing negative messages through techniques such as role-playing, modeling, and homework assignments is essential to introduce any new behaviors and to eliminate anxiety in the performance of existing skills.

Cognitive-behavioral approaches to assertiveness training have proven effective in improving social skills of elderly institutionalized patients (Berger & Rose, 1977). Combinations of modeling, role-playing, and other behavioral techniques with lectures and discussions have proven effective in improving interpersonal skills, increasing the rate and range of social interactions, producing desirable emotional changes, increasing the ability to make requests, and diminishing social anxiety in college students (Tigerman & Kassinove, 1977; Royce, 1976; Janda & Rimm, 1977). Also, Carlson (1976) found that combined cognitive and behavioral assertiveness training of student nurses resulted in more assertive behaviors and increased self-concept and self-acceptance. Although studies generally compare cognitive-behavioral assertiveness training to placebo controls or no-treatment groups, Tigerman and Kassinove (1976) found support for cognitive and behavioral treatments over behavioral treatment of nonassertive college students. It would be expected that teaching nurses to discriminate among aggressive, assertive, and nonassertive behaviors, identifying their rights and the rights of others, reducing the irrational beliefs and attitudes that interfere with assertiveness, and developing and practicing assertive skills would lead to behavior changes in terms of relationships, personal development, and system maintenance, dimensions that have been associated with favorable ward atmosphere.

The preponderance of attention to ward climate has centered around psychiatric wards. Recent interest, as cited above, has extended to some other long-term care wards or special care wards such as psychiatric, cancer, and dialysis units. The interpersonal skills involved in producing favorable ratings of ward atmosphere on psychiatric wards appear also related to better atmospheres on cancer, renal, and intensive care units. To extend the findings of ward atmosphere studies, the present investigation considered the spinal cord injury unit, a type of care facility not previously explored. Spinal cord injured patients share a number of characteristics with psychiatric, cancer, and dialysis patients. Spinal cord injured patients are long-term and, therefore, exposed to the ward for prolonged periods. Patients on a spinal cord injury ward require rehabilitation to daily living and, ideally, to employment just as psychiatric patients do. Spinal cord injured patients and psychiatric patients alike are often concerned about being perceived differently by others and rely on interactions with staff to gain practice in new roles. In addition, rehospitalization constitutes a major obstacle to rehabilitation, just as it does on psychiatric wards. Further, the especially unfortunate situations of spinal cord injured patients provide an ideal setting for an investigation of ward atmosphere. Spinal cord injured patients are highly dependent upon ward staff for care beyond the medical attention required on many medical wards (Eisenberg & Falconer, 1978). Dependency for care is also characteristic of cancer units, dialysis units, and intensive care units; however, in most cases, alert patients are able to attend to some of their own care such as feeding, bathing, and elimination. Given the similarities, it would seem likely that the dimensions that effect psychiatric, dialysis, cancer, and intensive care units would also effect spinal cord injured patients. It is possible that the nature of the spinal cord injured patient's dependence on ward staff might amplify the effects experienced by other patients.

In addition, there is more than one type of spinal cord injured patient. The differences in disability involved in paraplegia compared to quadriplegia provide a gradation in the difficulty of the rehabilitation process and the degree of dependence on nursing staff. Quadriplegia results from an injury or disease of the spinal cord that effects nerve integrity at the level involved in control and sensation to the arms. Quadriplegic patients are paralyzed in all four extremities and require bowel and bladder care. Paraplegia involves the spinal cord at a level below that serving the arms and, depending upon the level, may retain bowel and/or bladder control. Quadriplegics are essentially dependent on ward staff for all activities of daily living, e.g. mobility, dressing, bowel and bladder care. Paraplegics, on the other hand, can more easily make transfers, dress and feed themselves, and they are able to assist in their own bowel and bladder care (Rustad, 1975). It would seem that quadriplegic patients are more dependent on the ward and might, therefore, be more sensitive than paraplegic patients to any changes in ward atmosphere.

In summary, favorable social climates have been shown to be associated with positive outcomes on hospital wards such as rehabilitation, longer community stays, faster discharge rates, and fewer returns to hospitals. In the course of efforts to identify the elements of the more favorable social climates, the factors of relationship, personal development, and system maintenance have emerged. Elements of the factors related to positive ward outcomes appear to be appropriate results of cognitive-behavioral approaches to assertiveness training. It would seem, therefore, that the ward climate would be likely to alter as a function of assertiveness training of the caretakers of an environment. In addition, the perception of change is likely to be a function of the degree of dependency that an individual has on that environment.

Specifically, the present study investigated whether the patient's perception of his ward climate with respect to the dimensions of relationship, personal development, and system maintenance varies as a function of assertiveness training of his nurses. Assertiveness training followed a cognitive-behavioral approach that included teaching discrimination among assertive, aggressive, and nonassertive behaviors, identifying nurses rights and the rights of others, reducing nurses irrational beliefs and attitudes that might interfere with behaving assertively and practicing assertive skills. And, finally, the present investigation examined the effects of assertiveness training on the patients' perceptions of their nurses' interpersonal behavior in order to assess changes in positive and negative statements, "small talk," "feeling talk," problem-solving ability, anxiety in self-expression, and clarity of communications.

It was hoped that the results of the present study would provide direction and guidance in the care of spinal cord injured patients so that their stay in the hospital might be as comfortable as possible so that optimum support and control might be offered for the difficult task of rehabilitation.

METHODS

Subjects

All nursing personnel and patients on the spinal cord injury unit at Cleveland VA Hospital were included in the present investigation. Nursing staff included head nurses, registered nurses, licensed practical nurses, and nursing assistants. A total of seventy-three nursing personnel were involved. The nursing staffs of the two wards were alike with respect to age, education, race, and sex. The patients in the present study included both paraplegic and quadriplegic patients from both wards of the spinal cord injury unit, providing a total of forty-eight subjects. Patients who had been injured less than six months were excluded, since their care during this period typically differs from that of other patients. Similarly, a group of patients who had remained on the unit for several years due to the unavailability or inadequacy of post-hospital facilities were also excluded. The thirty-two remaining individuals on the two wards (sixteen on each ward) were alike insofar as possible with respect to age, education, race, marital status, duration of current admission, and degree of paralysis, i.e. paraplegia or quadriplegia.

Setting

The present investigation was conducted at Cleveland Veterans Administration Medical Center, a general medical-surgical care facility. Specifically, the investigation was carried out on the spinal cord injury unit. The spinal cord injury unit at CVAMC is a regional facility serving eight states. The spinal cord injury unit is divided into two wards, equivalent in size and staffing patterns. Assignment of nursing staff is to one ward or the other so that nursing staff is not shared by the two wards.

Measures

A modification of the Ward Atmosphere Scale (Weiss, 1975; Moos, 1968) was employed to assess the ward climate as perceived by the patients. The Ward Atmosphere Scale has shown good test-retest reliability and the original WAS has been shown to be valid when correlated with drop-out rates, release rates, and community tenures for psychiatric samples (Moos, 1975).

In addition, the present investigator devised the Nurses Interpersonal Index, a ten-item, self-report scale in order to measure behavior change in nurses following assertiveness training. Several measures of reliability of this instrument were calculated, all yielding high reliability coefficients.

Procedures

Two questionnaires were administered to patients on both wards: (1) the Ward Atmosphere Scale and (2) the Nurses Interpersonal Index. Both questionnaires were administered at two points: (1)

prior to the first assertiveness training session of nursing staff and (2) following the conclusion of the five sessions.

In order to assure that there were no effects resulting from the earlier measurement, Solomon's four-group design was employed (Solomon & Lessac, 1968). Half of the paraplegic patients and half of the quadriplegic patients on each ward were randomly selected and were administered initial testing. The remaining one-half of the patients in all groups were tested only at the conclusion of the study along with the patients who received initial testing.

Nursing personnel, in groups of three to five, from one of two spinal cord injury wards received five sessions of cognitive-behavioral assertiveness training. Training consisted of an introduction to the principles of assertiveness training, an examination of problems as perceived by trainees, elicitation of preconceived attitudes and personal values and attitudes that might interfere with assertive communications, and skills training. Skills training entailed the use of modeling, covert and overt behavior rehearsal, role reversal, and shadowing. All techniques were followed with feedback from the trainer and other trainees. Assertiveness training sessions occurred over a five-week period with one session per group per week. One and one-half hour sessions were held for each shift during the regular hours of the shift.

Nursing personnel from the opposite spinal cord injury ward received a comparable time listening to structured lectures on psychological subjects. Provisions were made to offer assertiveness training to the placebo group at the conclusion of this investigation.

RESULTS

The purpose of the present investigation was to determine whether perceived ward atmosphere and the perception of the interpersonal characteristics of nursing staff changed over time as a result of nurses having been given assertiveness training. Each patient provided (at a single test session) two scores: (1) a score on the Ward Atmosphere Scale and (2) a score for the Nurses Interpersonal Index. The Ward Atmosphere Scale was calculated as a total score of the profile scale scores ordinarily used. The total of the Ward Atmosphere Scale yielded a raw score that varied from a minimum of zero to a maximum of ninety-six. The Nurses Interpersonal Index was obtained by summing the scores for the five nurses rated by each patient, yielding a total score which could vary from a minimum of fifty to a maximum of three hundred.

The variables considered were (1) whether nurses received assertiveness training or were in the placebo control group, (2) whether patients were paraplegic or quadriplegic, (3) at what point in the program the measures were collected, before or after training, and (4) whether the patient had been administered pretesting.

Inspection of the means in Table 14-I indicates that none of the means on the Ward Atmosphere Scale differ appreciably from each other. In other words, assertiveness training of nursing personnel does not appear to have altered patients' perceptions of their ward atmosphere. Similarly, examination of Table 14-II reveals that

TABLE 14-I. MEAN SCORES AND STANDARD DEVIATIONS ON THE WARD ATMOSPHERE SCALE (N=4 per group)

Type of training	Type of injury	Tested or not tested	Pre-training	Post-training
Assertiveness	Paraplegia	pre-tested	M 214.50 SD 38.34	M 233.00 SD 31.86
		no pre-test		M 225.75 SD 49.18
	Quadriplegia	pre-tested	M 210.25 SD 30.66	M 139.50 SD 27.69
		no pre-test		M 229.00 SD 22.11
Placebo	Paraplegia	pre-tested	M 217.00 SD 36.81	M 221.25 SD 46.86
		no pre-test		M 214.25 SD 45.75
	Quadriplegia	pre-tested	M 225.00 SD 22.77	M 221.00 SD 39.35
		no pre-test		M 238.25 SD 27.52

TABLE 14-II. MEAN SCORES AND STANDARD DEVIATIONS ON THE NURSES INTERPERSONAL INDEX (N=4 per group)

Type of training	Type of injury	Tested or not tested	Pre-training	Post-training
Assertiveness	Paraplegia	pre-tested	M 46.00 SD 11.66	M 46.00 SD 9.76
		no pre-test		M 61.00 SD 13.64
	Quadriplegia	pre-tested	M 48.60 SD 6.03	M 51.50 SD 8.54
		no pre-test		M 54.50 SD 7.42
Placebo	Paraplegia	pre-tested	M 51.00 SD 12.73	M 53.75 SD 7.42
		no pre-test		M 50.50 SD 12.18
	Quadriplegia	pre-tested	M 43.25 SD 19.35	M 41.50 SD 23.30
		no pre-test		M 52.75 SD 7.18

scores on the Nurses Interpersonal Index do not differ noticeably from each other. It also appears that spinal cord injured patients do not perceive the interpersonal skill of their nurses to have altered as a result of assertiveness training. To confirm these impressions, three analyses were performed on each measure.

The first analyses, 2 (type of training) x 2 (type of injury) two-way ANOVA, showed that patients did not differ among themselves in perceptions of their ward atmosphere or their nurses interpersonal skill prior to training of ward nurses. These analyses also demonstrated that paraplegic patients did not differ from quadriplegic patients in their perceptions before training began.

The second analyses were performed to rule out interactions between pretesting effects and experimental treatments. A 2 (type of training) x 2 (type of injury) x 2 (pretest or no pretest) three-way ANOVA offered assurance that pretesting of patients did not effect final scores on the Ward Atmosphere Scale or the Nurses Interpersonal Index.

The third analyses compared the means of the Ward Atmosphere Scale scores and the Nurses Interpersonal Index scores at pretraining (left-hand column of Tables 14-I and 14-II) with the means of post-training scores of those groups receiving pretesting (right-hand column, Tables 14-I and 14-II). Scores were entered into a 2 (type of training) x 2 (type of injury) x 2 (time of testing) three-way ANOVA with repeated measures on the last factor. The apparent lack of change in patients' perceptions over time was confirmed by the analyses.

In summary, assertiveness training was offered to the nursing staff of one ward of a spinal cord injury unit while nurses on a comparable ward were in placebo control groups. It had been expected that assertiveness training would improve both quadriplegic and paraplegic patients' perceptions of their ward atmosphere and their nurses interpersonal skills. It was not clear whether or not differences would be found between paraplegic and quadriplegic patients, but it was felt that the increased physical dependence of quadriplegic patients on their nurses might effect perceptions differentially. As a review of the statistical analyses has shown, assertiveness training did not effect either patients' perceptions of their nurses assertiveness or their perception of the ward atmosphere.

On the other hand, correlation coefficients calculated between the Ward Atmosphere Scale and the Nurses Interpersonal Index demonstrated that a modest relationship ($r = .42$) exists between the two scales, suggesting that ward atmosphere is related to nurses' assertiveness.

DISCUSSION

The hypothesis that spinal cord injured patients' perceptions of the interpersonal characteristics of nursing staff and the perception of their ward atmosphere would change over time as a result of nurses having been given assertiveness training was not supported by the present results. The question of whether quadriplegic or paraplegic patients might detect changes in their ward environment differentially as a function of the degree of disability and dependency on nursing staff could not be answered in the absence of change, but there was no evidence that the two types of patients differed in their perceptions of their wards. Since the reliability of the Nurses Interpersonal Index was demonstrated and the reliability of the Ward Atmosphere Scale had been established, the possibility that assertiveness of nurses was unrelated to patients' perceptions of their ward atmosphere was considered. However, it was shown that a moderate relationship existed. On the other hand, when assertiveness of nurses was manipulated, no change was found. The absence of change suggests that the relationship is not causal in this particular setting or that the training was not successful.

The findings that five sessions of assertiveness training workshops in which all nursing personnel of a spinal cord injury ward participated had no effect on the way nurses were perceived by patients or on perceptions of ward environment was unexpected. Previous research has indicated the efficacy of assertiveness training in producing outcomes that appear related to the dimensions of the Ward Atmosphere Scale. In a prior study of assertiveness training of nurses, the nurses' self-reports and subjective impressions were measured; however, patients and other staff members did not evaluate the change (Carlson, 1976). It is possible that patients did not perceive the same changes that nurses experienced. It is unfortunate that this study contained no evaluation of training by nursing staff.

If it is the case that there is some relationship between the assertiveness of nurses and patients' perception of ward atmosphere, as the results indicate, and, if ward nurses become more assertive as a result of training, it could be that patients' perceptions of nurses have become relatively fixed after some interval. In some respects, relationships between nursing personnel and patients on a spinal cord injury unit approximate family relationships with respect to dependency and protracted duration, and roles may become somewhat fixed. It is possible that the changes sought by the assertive training workshops would not be perceived immediately.

On the other hand, Witkin (1976) observed increases in ratings of marital satisfaction using communication skills training in marital counseling cases. This investigation included both parties, however, and therapy was sought by the individuals receiving training. It is conceivable that the motivation of marriage partners, particularly those seeking counseling, may be greater than the motivation of nurses to increase patients' satisfaction with their ward.

A major obstacle to involvement of nursing staff in the assertiveness training workshops was their perception that they had been selected as a "problem" group. Many of the nursing personnel raised objections to making changes when similar changes or concessions were not required of patients or physicians. Although the present investigator anticipated the problem of incentive for change and attempted to illustrate the gains for nurses in terms of improved morale in the work setting as well as a possibility of reduced demands on the part of patients, nurses continued to see patients as the only beneficiaries.

Casual observation suggests that other factors may have operated as well. The observations of the interviewer indicated that patients' perceptions of both interpersonal skills of their nurses and the ward atmosphere seemed to be related to their general satisfaction with life. While discrimination between individuals was reliable, patients appeared imperceptive of changes.

Many nurses participated enthusiastically and reportedly profited from the training. For example, a group of nursing assistants were successful in having staffing patterns altered to their specifications after frequent, more aggressive attempts had failed. Another nurse reported that she had been successful in reducing the amount of verbal abuse she received from patients. Evidence that effects were generalized to other environments was obtained when another nurse related that he enjoyed more satisfying interactions with his girlfriend. One nursing assistant who reported satisfaction with the workshop was given support for her impression by a patient's spontaneous testimonial to her change. Most of the modifications reported reflected behaviors that would be expected to directly affect the individual, however. Only a few nurses requested assistance in improving interactions with patients.

These observations suggest several directions for further investigation. For example, a study that included patients, physicians, nursing staff, and other ancillary ward personnel might prove more effective at dealing with interpersonal difficulties relevant to Ward Atmosphere. In addition, greater cost-effectiveness may be achieved by a preliminary assessment and screening of trainees.

Evaluation of assertiveness training or communication skills workshops by trainees would provide some indication as to whether training was ineffective or whether patients failed to perceive any changes. Also, measurement of patients' perceptions of their ward staff at multiple points following assertiveness training would provide information concerning any delay in perception of change. Since it does appear that assertiveness of nurses is related to patients' perception of their ward atmosphere, it would appear that additional efforts aimed at modifying the assertiveness of nurses is warranted.

REFERENCES

Alberti, R. E., and Emmons, M. L. *Your Perfect Right.* San Luis Obispo: Impact Pubs. Inc., 1970.

Berger, R. M., and Rose, S. D. Interpersonal skills training with institutionalized elderly patients. *Journal of Gerontology,* 1977, *32,* 346-353.

Carlson, B. C. The effects of an assertion training group on the assertiveness of the self-concept of student nurses. Unpublished doctoral dissertation,

Cohen, J., and Struening, E. L. Opinions about mental illness: Hospital social atmosphere profiles and their relevance to effectiveness. *Journal of Consulting Psychology,* 1965, *38,* 291-299.

Corby, N. Assertion training with aged populations. *Counseling Psychologist,* 1975, *5,* 69-74.

Eisenberg, M. G., and Falconer, J. *Treatment of the Spinal Cord Injured: An Interdisciplinary Perspective.* Springfield, Illinois: Charles C Thomas, Publisher, 1979.

Eisler, R. M., Hersen, M., Miller, P. M., and Blanchard, E. B. Situational determinants of assertive behaviors. *Journal of Consulting and Clinical Psychology,* 1975, *43,* 330-340.

Ellis, A., and Harper, R. A. *A New Guide to Rational Living.* Englewood Cliffs, New Jersey: Prentice-Hall, Inc., 1975.

Flowers, J. V., & Booraem, C. D. Assertion training: The training of trainers. *Counseling Psychologist,* 1975, *5,* 29-36.

Hall, J. N. The content of ward rating scales for long-stay patients. *British Journal of Psychiatry,* 1977, *130,* 287-293.

Hay, D., and Oken, D. The psychological stresses of intensive care unit nursing. In R. H. Moos (Ed.), *Coping with Physical Illness*. New York: Plenum Medical Book Co., 1976.

Heimberg, R. G., Montgomery, D., Madsen, C. H., and Heimberg, J. S. Assertion training: A review of the literature. *Behavior Therapy*, 1977, *8*, 953-971.

Hersen, M., Eisler, R. M., Miller, P. M., Johnson, M. B., and Pinkston, S. G. Effects of practice, instructions, and modeling on components of assertive behavior. *Behavior Research and Therapy*, 1974, *12*, 295-310.

Jackson, J. Factors of the treatment environment. *Archives of General Psychiatry*, 1969, *21*, 39-45.

Janda, L. H., and Rimm, D. C. Type of situation and sex of counselor in assertive training. *Journal of Counseling Psychology*, 1977, *24*, 444-447.

Klagsbrun, S. C. Cancer, emotions, and nurses. *American Journal of Psychiatry*, 1970, *126*, 1237-1244.

Lange, A. J., and Jakubowski, P. *Responsible Assertive Behavior: Cognitive/Behavioral Procedures for Trainers*. Champaign, Illinois: Research Press, Co., 1976.

Linn, L. State hospital environment and rates of patient discharge. *Archives of General Psychiatry*, 1970, *23*, 346-351.

Moos, R. H. The differential effect of ward settings on psychiatric patients. *Journal of Nervous and Mental Diseases*, 1967, *145*, 272-283.

Moos, R. H. Situational analysis of a therapeutic community milieu. *Journal of Abnormal Psychology*, 1968, *73*, 49-61.

Moos, R. H. *Ward Atmosphere Scale, Preliminary Manual*. Stanford, California: Stanford University School of Medicine, 1969.

Moos, R. H. Differential effects of social atmospheres on psychiatric wards. *Human Relations*, 1970, *23*, 47-60.

Moos, R. H. Size, staffing, and psychiatric ward treatment environments. *Archives of General Psychiatry*, 1972, *26*, 414-418.

Moos, R. H. Changing the social milieus of psychiatric treatment settings. *Journal of Applied Behavioral Science*, 1973, *9*, 575-593.

Moos, R. H. Assessment and impact of social climate. In P. McReynolds (Ed.), *Advances in Psychological Assessment*. San Francisco: Jossey-Bass Publishers, 1975.

Moos, R. H., and Houts, P. Assessment of the social atmospheres of psychiatric wards. *Journal of Abnormal Psychology*, 1967, *73*, 595-604.

Nietzel, M. T., Martorano, R. D., and Melnick, J. The effects of covert modeling with and without reply training on the development and generalization of assertive responses. *Behavior Therapy*, 1977, *8*, 183-192.

Pierce, W. D., Trickett, E. J., and Moos, R. H. Changing ward atmosphere through staff discussions of the perceived ward environment. *Archives of General Psychiatry*, 1972, *26*, 35-41.

Rich, A. R., and Schroeder, H. E. Research issues in assertiveness training. *Psychological Bulletin*, 1976, *83*, 1084-1096.

Rimm, D. C., and Masters, J. C. *Behavior Therapy: Techniques and Empirical Findings.* New York: Academic Press, Inc., 1974.

Rosenthal, T. L., and Reese, S. L. The effects of covert and overt modeling on assertive behavior. *Behavior Research and Therapy*, 1976, *14*, 463-469.

Royce, W. S. Practice interactions, feedback and social skills training in the treatment of social inhibitions in friendship interactions. Unpublished doctoral dissertation.

Rustad, L. C. An investigation of the relationship between imaginational processes and motor inhibition: The fantasy life of paraplegics and quadriplegics. Unpublished doctoral dissertation, Case Western Reserve University, 1975.

Sarason, I. Verbal learning, modeling, and juvenile delinquency. *American Psychologist*, 1968, *23*, 254-266.

Scherer, S. E., and Freedberg, E. J. Effects of group videotape feedback on development of assertiveness skills in alcoholics: A follow-up study. *Psychological Reports*, 1976, *39*, 983-992.

Tigerman, S., and Kassinove, H. Effects on assertive training and cognitive components of rational therapy on assertive behaviors and interpersonal anxiety. *Psychological Reports*, 1977, *40*, 535-542.

Solomon, R. L., and Lessac, M. S. A control group design for experimental studies of developmental processes. *Psychological Bulletin*, 1968, *75*, 145-150.

Weiss, L. *Report on the study of emotional needs of the division of oncology at Good Samaritan Hospital.* Phoenix, Arizona: Good Samaritan Hospital, 1975.

Wolpe, J., and Lazarus, A. A. *Behavior Therapy Techniques:* New York: Pergamon Press, Inc., 1966.

Witkin, S. L. The development and evaluation of a group training program in communication skills for couples. Unpublished doctoral dissertation.

Zeichner, A., Wright, J. C., and Herman, S. Effects of situation on dating and assertive behavior. *Psychological Reports*, 1977, *40*, 375-381.

Chapter 15

STAFF AND PATIENT PERCEPTIONS OF THE REHABILITATION PROCESS

Dennis G. Stuart

Perhaps the most salient characteristic of a comprehensive rehabilitation program for the spinal cord injured is its social and technical complexity. Many different groups must work together to make the process function, each with its specialized vocabulary, training, techniques, and goals. Sophisticated medical services are necessary just to keep the newly injured patient alive and medically stable. The strengthening and retraining of remaining capacities requires skilled personnel and the need for social and psychological adjustment adds further problems. Rehabilitation nursing can be difficult because the patients are in the hospital for a period of months and may move from an almost helpless state to a mixture of dependency and independence that can be both frustrating and encouraging. Rehabilitation patients generally do not "walk out" of the hospital: they leave much improved but not cured, and this can cause dissatisfaction in some staff and some patients. In short, the rehabilitation hospital is a very lively social setting as well as a complex technical enterprise. Georgopolous (1972) has gone so far as to state that the organizational effectiveness of hospitals depends more on social efficiency than it does on technical-medical efficiency. This is perhaps even more true of the rehabilitation hospital than it is of the general hospital.

This research was supported in part by a grant from the Social and Rehabilitation Services Research and Training Center #4, Baylor College of Medicine.

I became familiar with the workings of a rehabilitation system while participating in a long-term project studying the behavior of spinal cord injured patients in an eighty-bed comprehensive rehabilitation center. Research team members worked closely with both staff and patients, and we were privy to a lot of gossip concerning problems between departments or between staff and patients or between supervisors and workers. Many of the problems seemed to be of a trivial nature, but there was an element in this type of discussion that seemed to be of more fundamental importance to the extent that it seemed to indicate a difference in philosophy about the rehabilitation process and the purpose of the hospital. I was sensitive to this issue because I was interested in studying the role of psychology in the in-patient treatment phase and was curious to learn how staff and patients viewed the relationships between the medical, physical, psychological, and social components of the program. In short, I wanted to develop a definition of what a rehabilitation center is all about from the people who inhabit it.

SOCIAL ECOLOGY

The business of asking people about their environment belongs to the domain of social ecology (Moos & Insel, 1974). A large number of instruments have been developed for a variety of settings: Moos (1974) developed the Ward Assessment Scale to describe psychiatric treatment programs and has modified versions for other types of settings. His scales define a relationship dimension, a personal development dimension, and a system maintenance dimension. It can be used to characterize a program, as a program evaluation device, or as a communications tool to increase consensus or spark discussion. Silbergeld, Koenig, Manderscheid, Meeker, and Hornung (1975) report a version of the Ward Assessment Scale for use with small therapy groups called the Group Atmosphere Scale. Jackson (1969) has developed the Characteristics of the Treatment Environment Scale to assess psychotherapeutic milieu. The Ward Evaluation Scale was developed by Rice, Klett, Berger, Sewall, and

Lemkau (1963) to describe the physical environment of psychiatric wards, the quality of services, and the patient management techniques used. Stern (1970) used the Murray (1938) Needs Press system to study colleges by comparing perceptions of the environment from the College Characteristics Index with student interests as reported on the Activities Index. Astin and Holland (1961) have also studied educational systems using their Environmental Assessment Technique.

All these methods attempt to get a description of an environment from the point of view of its inhabitants. This approach is well suited to health care and other service organizations because other measures of institutional functioning do not adequately describe all that is going on in service settings. A factory turning out bottle caps can measure output by a simple count. A surgical program might use number of deaths as its index of effectiveness, but a more complete evaluation would include measures of patient pain, length of hospitalization, and satisfaction with the treatment. Bottlecaps do not care what is done to them but people do, and process measures therefore become important.

Patients spend twenty-four hours a day in the hospital for a period of several weeks. Staff spend more than a third of their waking time at work and their satisfaction with their job and the work environment is an important characteristic of hospital functioning. In industry it has been found that job satisfaction is not strongly related to production but is related to staff turn-over, recruitment problems, and absenteeism (Atchinson & Lefferts, 1972; Friedlander, 1964; Patchen, 1960; Schneider & Snyder, 1975; Vroom, 1964). Smith, Kendall and Hulin (1969) describe employee satisfaction as an output variable; that is, producing satisfaction in employees is an important function of any organization that hopes to survive. Georgopolous and Massy (1962) found that health care professionals value job satisfaction as highly as salary, and Alutto, Hrebiniak, and Alonso (1971) found that programs that interfere with the professional-client relationship between nurses and patients have trouble hiring nurses even with competitive salaries.

Many organizational changes are made because of system demands rather than to simply improve output. Changes in staff assignments, supervisory practices, work rules, or physical structure often have little impact on outcome measures but do have an important influence on the way inhabitants view their environment. For instance, one of the *hot* issues at the Center was a debate about whether nurses and therapists should wear uniforms or street clothes while working. Considerable emotion was aroused over this issue and the arguments brought to light different philosophical positions about the nature of the rehabilitation process. The pro-uniform group espoused a medical model of treatment with clearly identified roles and responsibilities while the anti-uniform group preferred a kind of educational-social model that focused more on the interpersonal relationships between staff and patients. No one made a very convincing argument that simply doing away with uniforms would have any very great impact on the quality of rehabilitation experienced by patients, but there was a sense that it would matter in the day-to-day experience of both staff and patients.

All of this suggests that the perceptions inhabitants have of their environment are as important as objective measures of system performance. In one sense, perceptions may be more important than objective reality because the program elements are often shaped by what people think is happening rather than on reality. This is particularly true in service settings where it is difficult to get objective measures, or even agreement about what those measures should be.

Several goals were considered in developing a social ecological instrument for assessing rehabilitation programs. We wanted to know how well people in the program thought it was doing in providing the formal services of medical, physical, psychological, and social services. We wanted to know how they perceived the day-to-day operations of the system with reference to both the physical and social characteristics, and we wanted to know what people thought rehabilitation is all about—what the ingredients of a comprehensive rehabilitation program are. We were also curious to see if there was agreement among the various hospital groups on these questions, to see if there was a community of belief. Finally, we wanted to know what staff and patients thought about the role of psychological and social services in the overall process.

In addition to answering some questions about rehabilitation, we wanted to develop an instrument that would be useful to other rehabilitation workers as a descriptive, assessment and communications device. We felt that rehabilitation programs need a formal tool for assessing where they are and where they want to go, and for communicating this information to the hospital community in a systematic and nonthreatening manner.

None of the previously developed environmental assessment devices were suitable for a rehabilitation setting. Most were developed for psychosocial or educational programs and did not deal adequately with the medical and physical components and none provided a sufficiently detailed look at the many different staff groups and functions. This made it necessary to develop a new instrument.

INSTRUMENT DEVELOPMENT

The philosophy of development was to involve the hospital community and other rehabilitation professionals in all aspects of the project to increase the chance of creating a tool useful to rehabilitation workers. The first stage, therefore, consisted of a series of interviews with selected members of every major staff group in the hospital and with a number of ex-patients. Topics ranged from the availability of equipment to treatment philosophy. Out of these interviews came a set of interests and concerns that were then expressed in the form of a questionnaire with several hundred items. This questionnaire was taken back to the people interviewed for their critique and suggestions. A prototype instrument was then developed and piloted on a small group of staff and ex-patients. Their comments were used to develop the form that was administered to the hospital community: called the Rehabilitation Process Scales (RPS).

The RPS was presented in twelve sections with a total of 288 items. Various sections were factor analyzed after the data were collected to produce thirty factor scales defined by the items with high factor loadings on that scale. A second level factor analysis was also performed using the scale scores from the first level factors. This grouped the thirty first level scales into eight areas of interest (the details of this procedure can be found in Stuart, 1977). After analysis, the results were presented to the hospital community in a series of feedback sessions with all the response groups. These sessions clarified many questions raised by the responses to the instrument and identified scales that were low in usefulness or interest to the hospital. The result was that many scales have been dropped, modified, or combined with others so that the instrument has been reduced in size.

Participants

The RPS was distributed to members of physical therapy (PT), occupational therapy (OT), and social work (SW); to registered nurses, nurse clinicians, and surgical staff (RN); aides and licensed vocational nurses (Aide); to the vocational unit (VOC); and to the heads of nontreatment departments such as maintenance, housekeeping, business, pharmacy and labs—this was called the management group (MAN). Research team members were asked to respond as were nursing students doing a rotation at the Center. Volunteer workers were also asked to participate so the views of all individuals involved in the treatment process would be known. Finally, all spinal cord injured patients who had been at the Center for six weeks or more (about half an average stay) were asked to participate. Participation by all groups was strictly voluntary: no administrative pressure of any kind was applied, although the administration did allow staff to complete forms on hospital time.

The response rate was between eighty percent and one hundred percent for all but a few groups. The Aide group had only an eighteen percent return, the RN group had a thirty-seven percent return, the volunteers had a twenty percent return, and the patients had a fifty-three percent return. There were about 120 aides and 70 RNs at the Center so nursing alone accounted for more than half the staff. Even with the low proportional return rate, Aides and RNs were the largest response groups. The low return from the Aides was disappointing but not unexpected. Many aides refused the task outright and others did not return forms after accepting them. Many were quite open in saying they saw no point in projects like this and mentioned other studies they had participated in that had had no noticeable outcome on hospital operations. It should be noted that the Center was frequently a site for research projects and there had been concern that the staff had been "studied out."

It proved difficult to engage the volunteers in the task, which was surprising since they seemed to have high motivation to help the hospital. There seemed to be a positive reluctance to evaluate the hospital or to step beyond the bounds of a narrowly defined role as "helper." The most common comment was that they knew nothing about the operation of the hospital despite the fact that they spent considerable time there. Patient nonresponders either said they did not know enough or that they did not want to spend the time on a task that would not further their own rehabilitation. A few patients were eliminated from the sample because of problems with English.

The Center sample consisted of 102 treatment staff, thirty-five members of nontreatment groups, and seventeen patients. In addition the RPS was administered to eleven patients and nine staff at a twenty-four-bed spinal cord unit in a nearby Veterans Administration hospital. All staff groups on the unit were represented, but only one of the seventeen aides and three of the eight nurses responded so that again nursing was represented by a small sample of its membership.

RESULTS

Figure 15-1 shows the results for eight of the first level factor scales grouped according to the second level factor structure. Mean ratings for the Center treatment staff and patients and the VA staff and patients are shown. The response format was a 7-point rating scale ranging from 1, indicating a negative evaluation to 7, indicating a very positive evaluation. Note that patients at both facilities tended to make more positive evaluations than staff and Center participants were generally less critical of their program than the VA groups were of theirs.

The most critical evaluations at both institutions were obtained on the two Environmental Quality scales: Hospital Organization and Patient Security. The first deals with scheduling, availability of

TABLE 15-I. PERCENTAGE OF MONEY ASSIGNED TO GROUPS OR SERVICES

Target Group	Center Staff	Center Patients	VA Staff	VA Patients	
Facilities	39	30	28	18	*b
Physicians	2	15	23	19	c
Research	6	7	6	37	c
Nursing	19	7	13	4	*b
Physical Therapy	7	20	4	4	*c
Recreation	11	7	4	3	
Occupational Therapy	5	7	5	4	
Social Work	4	0	11	3	*a,b
Vocational Services	4	4	4	2	
Psychology	3	2	2	4	

Two-way ANOVA:

* $p < .05$

  $p < .01$

a = between facilities

b = between staff and patients

c = interaction

equipment, and communications. The second asks if patients feel threatened by some staff members and if patients feel free to express their feelings about the hospital and staff. The responses are near the scale midpoint, indicating some ambivalence about the quality of day-to-day functioning. The higher ratings obtained for the Program Quality scales demonstrates the independence of judgments concerning the quality of program elements and environmental elements mentioned earlier. Presumably if scheduling difficulties were to get completely out of hand, or if equipment could not be found, then program quality would suffer. However, it is likely that a great deal of inefficiency and even frustration could be tolerated before serious effects would be noted in the quality of the rehabilitation "product." Administrators tend to know this either intuitively or from experience, so when the budget is tight it is the so-called "amenities," such as extra nursing care or newer equipment that gets cut. The effect is to reduce satisfaction with the environment without an immediate effect on outcomes. The longer term effects on staff morale and recruitment, or on referrals are not clear and are hard to demonstrate in any case.

The six areas of program functioning received very similar ratings from staff and patients at the Center but were related differently by VA staff and patients. The Supportive Staff scale asks about staff willingness to help patients with both physical and emotional support. The Patient Information and Patient Preparation scales deal with the information provided to patients and their families about the patients' condition and the operation of the hospital; and with the extent to which staff understand the needs of patients and their families and offer preparation to them for the patients' return home. The Rehabilitation Quality, Routine Care, and Critical Care scales ask how well the system delivers rehabilitation, nursing, and medical services. They cover the formal treatment characteristics of the program.

The discrepancy between the Patient Security and Supportive Staff ratings deserves some further comment. The feedback sessions made it clear that most respondents did indeed feel that staff were generally supportive of patients' needs. There was also agreement that there was a problem with a small number of staff who abused their position by threatening patients when they complained about the treatment they were receiving. This was understood to be primarily a supervision problem, although some staff felt it raised larger issues of staffing problems and hiring practices. Both staff and patients agreed the problem was primarily with the aide group and some staff argued for hiring more R.N.s and fewer aides, while administrators pointed out cost and recruitment difficulties.

In general then, Center staff and patients rated their program favorably with some problems noted in day-to-day functioning; VA patients were more critical of their program and the VA staff was the most critical of all response groups. It was possible to combine the Center staff treatment groups because their responses to these sections of the RPS were very similar. In fact, five response group clusters could be identified, characterized by how positive or critical their evaluations were across the various scales. The positive response cluster consisted of aides, patients, and volunteers. The aides were the most positive on virtually every section of the RPS. Patients and volunteers tended to be slightly more positive than treatment staff on most sections. The Center inpatient treatment staff formed the middle response cluster. Their evaluations were generally positive but usually lower than the first cluster. The RN group tended to be the most critical of the treatment groups. The vocational unit, research team, and the nursing students formed the critical response cluster, with the nursing students making the most negative ratings of any Center group. These three groups differed from one another from one section of the RPS to another but overall tended to be more critical than the treatment staff. VA patients and VA staff each formed distinct response groups as has already been noted. Statistically significant differences were found between the positive response cluster and the three critical response clusters with the Center Treatment staff falling between and not differing at a statistically significant level from either of the extreme clusters at the Center. Differences between the two facilities were generally significant as were staff/patient differences at the VA.

It was something of a surprise to get such positive ratings from patients and aides since the nonsystematic impression had been that there were a lot of complaints. The most troublesome possibility that suggested itself was that the sample was not representative. Patients, aides, and volunteers were all represented by a smaller proportion of their population than were most staff groups. It may have been that those with negative opinions refused the task. The RN group, on the other hand, was the most negative treatment group and had the smallest representation in the treatment staff cluster. There was no good way to resolve this question, and it must remain open. For this reason the aide group was not included with the other treatment staff, and likewise the volunteers were always analyzed as a separate group.

In the feedback sessions we asked people about these positive responses and learned that most participants felt the complainers were few in number, although quite loud and visible. Certain patients were noted for their negative reactions to the system, but most participants felt the actual count of dissatisfied patients was small. This, of course, did not resolve the sampling problem, but provided a plausible explanation for the phenomenon.

A second line of reasoning on this matter proceeded from the finding that staff employed a year or less were consistently more positive in their ratings than were staff employed more than a year. This difference was statistically significant for some scales and not others, but the direction of difference was always the same: new staff were less critical than experienced staff. This suggests that those who are less familiar with the functioning of the system tend to give it the benefit of the doubt—when they don't know about an area of hospital functioning they tend to rate it positively. This is an understandable bias in a culture that values health care services and activities and assigns them high status. Patients, volunteers, new staff, and also aides have little to do with the backstage functioning of the hospital, and their ratings of many program elements were based partly on experience and partly on what they thought or hoped might be happening. We were particularly struck by the faith (or hope) patients placed in the knowledge and skill of the staff. Ex-patients tended to be much more vocal about shortcomings in the staff and program. Of course hospitalized patients have little recourse but to trust staff, and it may be that for them to criticize the system too severely while still in it would be a very anxiety-producing activity. If this is true then it will be difficult to get a useful evaluation of the program from inpatients. The lower ratings obtained from VA patients, then, may be a function of the fact that some of them had been rehospitalized after living in the community, while almost all the Center patients were new admissions.

Talking with the nursing students and the research personnel who made the most critical ratings of the hospital suggested that their negative perceptions were due, in part, to a discrepancy between their understanding of what a rehabilitation program *should* be and what it actually was, combined with the fact that they had no responsibility for creating or maintaining the present system. It is also part of the function of students and researchers to be critical and to evaluate what they see against theory, whereas treatment staff are more oriented towards realities and day-to-day problems.

Intergroup Comparisons

The similarities in responses of the various treatment staff (and the management group) were somewhat surprising because part of the impetus for the study had been the perception of disagreement between the departments on hospital functioning. By and large these differences did not emerge on overall ratings of system performance. There were however, several sections of the RPS designed specifically to get at possible interdepartmental conflicts and differences in priorities. The most direct measure was the Intergroup Strain scale which asked respondents to rate the amount of strain or tension they feel between themselves and each of eighteen hospital groups on a scale from zero (no strain) to six (severe strain).

The majority of strain ratings were between zero and two, indicating a low overall level of interdepartmental tension. The ratings of treatment staff and patients fell between one and two while ratings of auxiliary or supportive services such as housekeeping or pharmacy were between zero and one. In fact, the rank-order correlation between the strain ratings and ratings of amount of intergroup contact as collected from the Contact scale was 0.89. Nursing, which occupies the most central position in the hospital in terms of contacting other groups, received the highest strain ratings from other staff: 2.07 for Aides and 1.89 for RNs. The highest strain rating was the 3.71 assigned by nursing students to the Aide group. The pattern of ratings at the two facilities suggest that ratings of zero are given only between groups with little or no contact while a level of one is the minimum expected for groups that work together. Levels of 2 or 3 indicate mild, but reducible tension levels while ratings of 4 or above should be taken by supervisors and administrative personnel as indicating the existence of a serious breakdown in interdepartmental communications and cooperation.

The low interdepartmental strain ratings were discussed in the feedback sessions and the consensus obtained was that the rank and file of most departments do not perceive much problem with other groups; but supervisors, who have to negotiate allocation of resources and resolve such interdepartmental disputes as do occur, do tend to see and rate a higher level of interdepartmental strain. The exception to this was in nursing where the rank and file tend to

Perceptions of Rehabilitative Process   255

perceive more tension. In the feedback sessions nurses tended to state that nursing services were neither properly understood nor valued by other treatment disciplines.

The priorities of the various response groups were assessed by three scales: Group Size, Money Distribution and Important Aspects of Rehabilitation. The first two presented respondents with a list of hospital groups or service areas. First they were asked to say whether each group should be increased in size, kept the same, or reduced. They were then asked to distribute a hypothetical $100,000 grant in any way they liked among the groups, with the purpose of improving patient services. The rank-order correlation coefficient between the Group and Money scales was +0.88, indicating considerable similarity in these two tasks. Nevertheless each scale illuminated slightly different aspects of the respondent's interests.

Only three services were judged to need expansion by fifty percent or more of Center staff: recreation, with an agreement of sixty-three percent; registered nurses (57%), and volunteers (51%). Patients did not agree that any service or group needed expansion; their highest agreement was for more volunteers (35%) but of course this means that 65 percent did not see this need. At the VA, 78 percent of the staff thought more volunteers were needed and fifty-six percent wanted more aides and physicians. VA patients also wanted more physicians (64%). At both facilities then, the need for expansion was seen in groups that deliver day-to-day patient care. Except for the need for MDs at the VA, most respondents seemed to be focusing on groups that help increase patient comfort rather than the therapy groups. This is consistent with the earlier finding that the quality of program elements is high, but environmental characteristics could be improved.

The money distribution presents a picture consistent with the Size scale but with some interesting features of its own: Table 15-I shows the mean percentage of money given by staff and patients at each facility to ten departments or areas of program functioning; a two-way analysis of variance between staff and patients and facilities was performed, and those areas with significant differences are indicated. The largest amounts were assigned to facilities, which included space, equipment, food, maintenance, and housekeeping activities. This is consistent with a concern for environmental quality, although equipment has treatment implications as well. Physicians received fairly large proportions from all groups but Center staff, who tended to focus more on nursing and recreation than did the other groups. Nursing was given more money by staff than by patients at both programs.

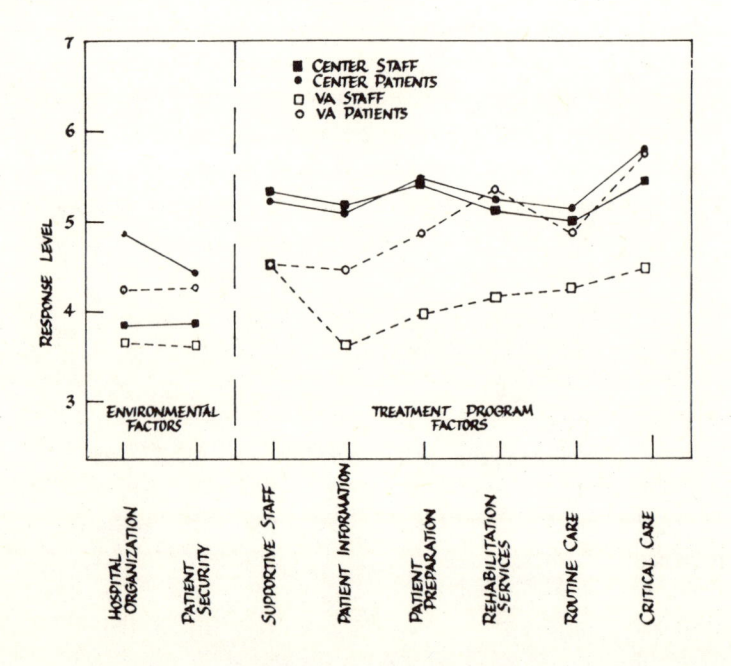

Figure 15-1. Results for eight of the first level factor scales grouped according to the second level factor structure.

VA patients, surprisingly, gave 34 percent of their money to research activities. Conversations with patients suggest this money would be intended for medical research into a *cure* for spinal cord injury, or at least for better electromechanical aids to mobility. Center patients, on the other hand, gave their second-largest amount to physical therapy, which suggests a difference in outlook between the two patient populations. Note that patients differ from staff on many of these categories.

Relatively small amounts were assigned to the last five categories, which include all the nonmedically oriented therapies. Occupational therapy comes the closest to the medical-physical treatment model but is often seen by staff and patients as a recreational or educational activity, an image that the occupational therapists have been attempting to alter for some time. The mean percentages assigned to the psychosocial and vocational activities fall below even recreation. This strongly suggests that these activities are not seen as very central to the business of the hospital, or to the process of rehabilitation; whereas medical interventions, nursing, and physical therapy are. It is not surprising to find this result in a medical setting such as a hospital, but it does raise once again the question of the proper role for the psychosocial services in such settings.

In discussing these results with staff and patients the following points were made: (1) many people are not sure what psychologists and social workers do; (2) staff have some doubts about how effective psychosocial workers are. This concern often arises when the staff try to define the psychologist or social worker as one who is supposed to "calm" troublesome patients while the worker is attempting to define a longer-term, programmatic, rehabilitation role; (3) many patients resent the implication that they are "crazy" or need help adjusting; and (4) patients are so busy with the physical and medical programs that there is little time left for other types of interventions. At the Center, for instance, there is no space set aside for either individual or group counseling and attempts to run such programs on the wards interfere with nursing routines. Both staff and patients agreed there were occasional patients who needed psychological counseling or therapy, but many patients felt such services were not relevant to their needs.

Interestingly, the last section of the RPS showed that patients *were* interested in psychosocial issues, if not in psychosocial treatment. The Important Aspects of Rehabilitation section asked respondents to list the ten things they thought were most important in a person's rehabilitation. Things listed might be people, philosophies, programs, devices, or whatever. The responses were coded into a small set of categories by several raters. Table 15-II shows the percentages of responses obtained in each category for the major response groups.

TABLE 15-II. IMPORTANT ASPECTS OF REHABILITATION: PERCENTAGE RESPONSES

Response Category	Center Staff	Center Patients	VA Staff	VA Patients
Physical/Medical Services	15	30	22	30
Patient Characteristics	11	20	21	14
Family/Community Attitudes*	9	15	4	16
Staff Attitudes	9	3	17	4
Psychosocial Services	8	6	5	11
Post-Hospital Programs	8	5	2	7
Patient/Family Involvement in Planning	10	2	8	0
Hospital Organization	11	1	6	1
Recreation	5	5	5	4
Facilities	7	3	5	3
Miscellaneous	9	10	5	10
	100	100	100	100

* Chi^2, $p < .05$

† Chi^2, $p < .01$

All groups most frequently mentioned the formal program elements of physical and medical treatment; however, the second most frequent items dealt with patient characteristics such as intelligence, personality, and motivation. For patients, family and community attitudes were next most often mentioned, and in fact, the first three categories account for 60 to 65 percent of the patient responses. Staff, on the other hand, saw staff attitudes as more important than did patients, with the VA staff particularly concerned with this area. Staff also saw patient and family involvement in planning the rehabilitation program as more important than did patients. Center staff were more concerned with hospital organization and the selection and training of skilled staff than were other groups.

Psychosocial and vocational services appear higher in the ranking on this task while facilities and recreation appear lower than they did in other sections. To reconcile these differences, it might be hypothesized that the hospital community would like to have better facilities and recreation programs but do not think these are of great importance in the rehabilitation process. Psychosocial programs, on the other hand, are seen as moderately important but are not seen as needing expansion.

Staff and patients tend to agree on the importance of the medical-physical program elements and on the importance of patient characteristics. They differ in that patients are more concerned with the attitudes and reactions of family, friends, and community while staff focus on program characteristics and staff attitudes. This division of interest makes sense and is healthy in that it is staff who must create and maintain the treatment program and patients who live in the community. Problems might arise only if the two groups do not realize that their priorities may be slightly different.

The category "post-hospital programs" appears in this section of the instrument for the first time—mentioned by a few staff and patients. This highlights the fact that this study surveyed only one type of rehabilitation program: the in-patient, comprehensive treatment facility which accepts newly injured patients. Those in a transitional living program or outpatient facility might very well make a different ranking of priorities. The strong emphasis on medical-physical treatment is appropriate for newly injured patients. If we accept the responses of the professionals and patients studied here, the difficult and complex task of saving patient lives and maximizing physical functioning is being well handled by the existing programs. These staff and patients see little need to change the present structure, except to make the environment a little more comfortable and efficient. There are a few radicals in the hospital decrying the medical model and demanding stronger social or psychosocial programs. And yet, it is still argued that the psychosocial adjustment to a severe physical disability is difficult and that there is a role for treatment programs in this area.

It may be that this argument makes more sense when phrased as a sequencing issue rather than a matter of priorities; that is, we should ask *when* are psychosocial programs most useful, rather than asking which elements of the rehabilitation process are most useful. It then makes sense to say that psychosocial treatment belongs to the post-hospital treatment phase, beginning with the transition period as the patient prepares to leave the hospital. If this separation of program functions is made, then many of the problems in integrating psychosocial treatment programs with medical goals and techniques disappear. Once out of the medical setting, these programs can then define their own goals without fear that they will conflict with the strenuous demands placed on staff and patients intent on the task of maximizing physical functioning.

Many patients plan to "walk out" of the hospital and it takes time for them to learn that this will not happen. Patients worry about the reactions of family and friends to their disability and they wonder what they will and will not be able to do. During hospitalization however, most patients are not willing or able to deal constructively with these fears and worries. It is fairly common for patients to focus on their physical rehabilitation activities as a way of dealing with their anxieties. They want to know how much functional return they will have before investing a lot of thought about the future. Patients have mentioned frequently how exhausted they sometimes get from the physical exercises—they have little excess energy to use for planning the future, particularly when the conditions that will shape the future are still unclear. I do not see this as a form of resistance or an unwillingness to face facts. I see it as taking first things first. Eventually patients will have to deal with a known physical and social situation, and it is at that point that psychological intervention can be useful and productive. Exactly when this will occur will vary from patient to patient and from program to program, but as a general rule it will be late in the hospitalization, or after the person has returned to the community.

The linkage of psychosocial treatment with the medical program has seemed to make sense from the point of view of coordinating planning and centralizing services. Funding has been easier to obtain for medical services and psychosocial programs have been tacked-on to the hospitalization period in order to bring them under the funding umbrella. It has also been argued that early intervention can help patients make a faster and smoother adjustment. Hospital staff have also wanted psychologists or psychiatrists available to deal with "problem" patients (those who do not cooperate with the program), and it has seemed natural to combine this system's maintenance activity with an attempt to deliver psychosocial rehabilitation services.

My experience has been that in-hospital psychosocial programs are difficult to integrate with hospital routines, that early intervention is not as efficient as properly timed intervention, and that psychosocial treatment goals are not readily obtained while the person is in a medical treatment setting. I was curious, therefore, to see if staff and patients would perceive any weaknesses in psychosocial services, or if they would suggest any expansion. The relatively high level of satisfaction and moderate importance assigned to the area was not surprising, however, and helped to bring into focus the importance of the sequencing issue.

EPILOGUE

The RPS has been reduced in size and restructured somewhat as a result of the data collected in this study. It is intended for use by comprehensive rehabilitation programs as a monitoring, assessment, and communications device. As a monitoring device it can warn administrators or supervisors when program elements are not functioning well or when interdepartmental tensions are rising. As an assessment tool it provides a way to measure the effects of program changes on staff and patient perceptions; and as a communications device it is useful in letting the hospital community know what the various departments and groups are thinking. Bowers (1973) found that feedback of survey results is one of the most powerful techniques for improving organizational functioning. The discussion of survey results provides a focus and starting point for needed changes and a medium that allows participants to make their feelings known without jeopardizing their position or threatening someone else's position. Surveys do cost time and money and the feedback sessions may raise more questions than can be answered, so any organization must weigh the costs and benefits of an evaluation. However, rehabilitation settings, with their many disciplines, complex goals, and dense social structure can learn much from such evaluations.

REFERENCES

Alutto, J. A., Hrebiniak, L. G., and Alonso, R. C. Variations on hospital employment and influence perceptions among nursing personnel. *Journal of Health and Social Behavior, 12,* 38-44, 1971.

Astin, A. W., and Holland, J. L. The environmental assessment technique: A way to measure college environments. *Journal of Educational Psychology, 52,* 308-315, 1961.

Atchinson, T. J., and Lefferts, E. A. The prediction of turnover using Hertzberg's job satisfaction technique. *Personnel Psychology, 25,* 53-64, 1972.

Bowers, D. G. "OD Techniques" and their results in 23 organizations: The Michigan ICL study. *Journal of Applied Behavioral Science, 9,* 21-43, 1973.

Friedlander, F. Job characteristics or satisfiers or dissatisfiers. *Journal of Applied Psychology, 48,* 388-392, 1964.

Georgopoulos, B. S. (Ed.). *Organization Research on Health Institutions.* Ann Arbor, Michigan: Institute for Social Research, University of Michigan, 1972.

Georgopoulos, B. S., and Massy, F. C. *The community general hospital.* New York: Macmillan Co., 1962.

Jackson, J. Factors of the treatment environment. *Archives of General Psychiatry, 21,* 39-45, 1969.

Moos, R. H. *Evaluating Treatment Environments.* New York: John Wiley & Sons, Inc., 1974.

Moos, R. H., and Insel, P. M. (Eds.). *Issues in Social Ecology.* Palo Alto, California: National Press Books, 1974.

Murray, H. *Explorations in Personality.* New York: Oxford University Press, 1938.

Patchen, M. Absence and employee feelings about fair treatment. *Personnel Psychology, 13,* 349-360, 1960.

Rice, C. E., Klett, S. L., Berger, D. G., Sewall, L. G., and Lemkau, P. V. The ward evaluation scale. *Journal of Clinical Psychology, 19,* 251-258, 1963.

Schneider, B., and Synder, R. A. Some relationships between job satisfaction and organizational climate. *Journal of Applied Psychology,* 1975, *60,* 318-328.

Silbergeld, S., Koenig, G. R., Manderscheid, R. W., Meeker, B. F., and Hornung, C. Assessment of environment-therapy systems: The group atmosphere scale. *Journal of Consulting and Clinical Psychology, 43,* 460-469, 1975.

Smith, P. C., Kendall, L. M., and Hulin, C. L. *The Measurement of Satisfaction in Work and Retirement.* Chicago: Rand McNally, 1969.

Stern, G. G. *People in Context.* New York: John Wiley & Sons Inc., 1970.

Stuart, D. G. Development of a survey instrument assessing staff and patient perceptions of comprehensive rehabilitation programs. Unpublished doctoral dissertation, University of Houston, 1977.

Vroom, V. H. *Work and Motivation.* New York: John Wiley & Sons, Inc., 1964.

Appendix

Opening Remarks made at the Sixth Annual Conference on The Care and Treatment of the Spinal Cord Injured
November 2-3, 1978, Park Plaza Hotel, Cleveland, Ohio

Paul M. Cheremeta
National Vice President, Paralyzed Veterans of America

On behalf of President Joe Romagnano and the Officers and Staff of the Paralyzed Veterans of America it is my pleasure to welcome you to the Sixth Annual Conference on the Care and Treatment of the Spinal Cord Injured.

Joe would very much like to be with us today but he is attending a meeting of the Technological Research Foundation of the PVA in Washington, D.C. I'll explain the coincidence as well as the significance of this occurrence later.

This is the third conference to be co-sponsored by the Buckeye Chapter of PVA, a chapter of which I am especially proud, being both a past president and current member.

I am often asked what PVA is and what we do. If I have a willing listener and the time I can usually launch myself into a half hour discussion and still not cover everything. A brief scanning of the literature in your packet including the *Paraplegia News*, our official publication, will give you an idea of some of the things our organization does. You will find that we are into many things such as spinal cord injury research, civil rights advocacy, legislation, employment, and barrier free design for both veteran and nonveteran catastrophically disabled individuals.

I like to think of PVA as one of the very few associations that can truly call itself a consumer organization. To me the terminology "consumer organization," or "consumer group," "group of consumers," and the like, while very much in vogue, is also very often misused. We are all consumers of many things. As an obvious example I would venture to guess that nearly 100 percent of the people in this room, including those in wheelchairs, drive a motor vehicle. Some of us may be unfortunate enough to own Firestone® 500 steel belted tires or Ford™ Pintos, yet I do not think we will see many groups of Firestone or Ford owners sprouting up all over the country. Nor do I foresee large scale participation in consumer health organizations, although so-called consumer activists and even the federal government try to push us in this direction. Most of us simply do not feel enough of a common bond to form or participate in a true grass roots consumer organization.

Perhaps the devastating effects of disease or trauma to the spinal cord creates a different situation. Shortly after World War II a gutsy group of Veterans banded together to demand and receive the care and rehabilitation they so rightly deserved. Their efforts resulted in specialized Spinal Cord Injury units in the Veterans Administration Hospitals and finally in many civilian centers as well. More than thirty years later we are still fighting to improve the quality of the care and treatment we receive.

As a true consumer organization, all PVA members are paralyzed. All are veterans. This includes our officers, our Executive Director, and most of our National Office staff. It also includes our corps of Service Officers throughout the country who handle cases of all veterans with skill, expertise, and most importantly, compassion.

As I mentioned, PVA has many facets; it does a lot of things. Today our focus is on communication and continuing education of the health care professionals in the many fields that are involved in the rehabilitation of the spinal cord injured.

I mentioned that our National President would be here today were he not in a meeting of our Technological Research Foundation. Today he will participate in the review of research proposals to determine their merits. During this fiscal year alone PVA will fund projects in the amount of $300,000 based on their scientific merit alone.

I know we are dedicated to improving our lives and the lives of others. We hope you are too. On behalf of the members of PVA we hope you have a meaningful and rewarding experience.

AUTHOR INDEX

Ablin, A. R. 189, 202
Adams, E. 21, 34
Agulera, D. C. 100, 106
Akridge, R. L. 154, 169, 171
Alberti, R. E. 55, 56, 83, 89, 228, 240
Alby, J. M. 182, 202
Alby, N. 182, 191, 202
Alexander, L. 133, 147
Alonso, R. C. 245, 262
Alutto, J. A. 245, 262
Anthony, E. J. 202
Aradine, C. R. 178, 202
Arieti, S. 222
Astin, A. W. 245, 262
Atchinson, T. J. 245, 262
Axelrod, B. H. 191, 202

Barber, B. 30, 34
Barofsky, I. 137, 147, 148, 161, 170
Beavers, W. 174, 203
Beavin, J. 17, 27, 34
Berger, D. G. 244, 262
Berger, R. M. 229, 240
Bernard, L. F. vii, 112-127
Berne, E. 209
Birdwhistell, R. L. 103, 106
Blanchard, E. B. 226, 240
Bluebond-Langner, M. 174, 179, 181, 182, 188, 202
Booraem, C. D. 227, 240
Bowers, D. G. 89, 262
Bowers, S. 89
Braatan, R. 3, 14
Bradley, R. F. 111
Brown, B. 214, 221
Burton, L. 203

Cahn, J. 221
Cairns, N. V. 185, 203
Capelli, A. 163, 171
Carlin, H. 163, 171
Carlson, B. C. 227, 228, 240

Carpenter, J. O. 133, 147, 221
Carr, A. 202, 204
Cartwright, A. 20, 34
Castelnuovo, P. 132, 147
Chadwick, D. L. 176, 204
Cheremeta, P. M. 263-265
Christensen, D. B. 165, 170
Clapp, M. J. 174, 202
Cobb, A. B. 41, 56
Cohen, J. 225, 240
Cohn, G. L. 133, 147
Conger, J. J. 180, 203
Conroe, R. M. 153, 164, 170
Corby, N. 226, 240
Czaczkes, J. W. 133, 147

Davis, F. 111
Davis, J. E. 153, 156, 165, 171
Deasy, P. M. vii, 173-205
Delatuer, B. J. 221
Dell Orto, A. E. 42, 56
Dodge, J. S. 148, 170
Dziurbejok, M. 148, 161, 170

Easson, W. M. 177, 202
Eisenberg, M. G. vii, 41, 51, 56, 158, 159, 171, 231, 240
Eisler, R. M. 226, 227, 240, 241
Ellicott, E. 176, 204
Ellis, A. 154, 171, 229, 240
Emmons, M. L. 89, 228, 240
Epstein, C. 153, 156, 166, 171
Exline, R. V. 99, 100

Falconer, J. viii, 35-57, 51, 56, 231, 240
Feifel, H. 177, 202
Feigenbaum, H. 133, 147
Fensterheim, H. 89
Fink, S. 133, 147
Finkelstein, F. 133, 147
Flowers, J. V. 227, 240
Ford, C. V. 132, 147

267

Fordyce, W. E. 31, 34, 213, 221
Fowler, R. S. 221
Freedberg, E. J. 226, 227, 242
Friedlander, F. 245, 262
Friedman, S. B. 189, 203
Friedson, E. 67, 111
Fuerstein, R. C. 202
Futterman, E. J. 182, 183, 189, 202

Gaarder, K. 214, 221
Garrett, J. 41, 56
Georgopolous, B. S. 243, 245, 262
Ginott, H. G. 13, 14
Glock, C. Y. 177, 203
Goffman, E. 67, 93, 101, 106
Goggin, I. 12, 14
Goldberg, G. 67
Goldenson, R. M. 42, 56
Gordon, T. 13, 14
Gossett, J. 174, 203
Gottlieb, H. 23, 24
Gotz, V. 163, 171
Grollman, E. A. 177, 203
Guyer, E. G. 6, 14

Hall, E. T. 92, 93, 95, 96
Hall, J. N. 225, 240
Hallenbeck, P. N. 133, 147
Hansen, Y. 178, 203
Hanson, R. W. 156, 164, 171
Harper, R. A. 240
Hartman, G. 204
Hassanein, R. 185, 203
Hay, D. 44, 56, 225, 241
Heimberg, J. S. 226, 228, 241
Heimberg, R. G. 226, 227, 228, 241
Henley, N. J. 93, 94, 97, 101, 106
Henry, J. 26, 34
Herman, S. 226, 242
Hersen, M. 226, 227, 240, 241
Hersh, S. 12, 14
Hinton, J. 152, 171
Hofer, M. A. 189, 203
Hoffman, I. 30, 34, 182, 183, 189, 202
Hohmann, G. W. 153, 156, 165, 171
Holland, J. L. 245, 262
Holmes, T. 190, 204
Hornung, C. 244, 262
Hostler, S. L. 177, 203

Houts, P. 225, 241
Howarth, R. 182, 203
Hrebiniak, L. G. 245, 262
Hulka, B. S. 151, 162, 163, 171
Hulin, C. L. 245

Imboden, J. B. 222
Insel, P. M. 244, 262

Jackson, D. 17, 27, 34
Jackson, E. N. 177, 203
Jackson, J. 225, 241, 244, 262
Jakubowski, P. 85, 89, 226, 227, 228, 229, 241
Janda, L. H. 227, 230, 241
Janis, I. L. 148, 171
Johnson, M. B. 227, 241
Jourard, S. M. 101, 106

Kagan, J. 180, 203
Kantor, D. 174, 203
Kaplan-Denour, A. 133, 147
Kard, T. 176, 189, 204
Kardinal, C. G. 152, 159, 172
Karon, M. 174, 179, 188, 204
Kassinove, H. 226, 230, 242
Kastenbaum, R. 177, 189, 203
Katz, E. R. 175, 200, 203
Kellerman, J. 175, 200, 203, 204
Kendall, L. M. 245
Kendon, A. 99
Kerr, N. viii, 107-111
Kiely, W. 18, 34
King, S. H. 67
Kitsen, J. 133, 147
Klagsbrun, S. C. 44, 56, 225, 241
Kleck, R. 94
Kleiber, N. 161, 171
Klett, S. L. 244, 262
Koenig, G. R. 244, 262
Koocher, G. P. 174, 203
Koupernik, C. 183, 202, 295
Krall, L. P. 111
Kubler-Ross, E. 154, 171
Kung, F. 177, 183, 190, 193, 204
Kutscher, A. 202, 204

Lange, A. J. 226, 227, 228, 241
Lansky, S. B. 174, 185, 203

Author Index

Larkin, J. C. 148, 161, 170
Lascari, A. D. 189, 204
Launier, R. 185, 191, 203
Lazarus, A. A. 227, 242
Lazarus, R. S. 185, 191, 203
Lecron, L. M. 192, 203
Lefferts, E. A. 245, 262
Lehmann, J. F. 221
Lehr, W. 174, 203
Lemkau, P. V. 245, 262
Lessac, M. S. 234, 242
Levin, L. 148, 171
Levine, E. 41, 56
Levy, N. B. 40, 56, 131, 147, 161, 171
Lewis, J. 174, 203
Light, L. 161, 171
Lindemann, C. A. 161, 171
Linn, L. 226, 241
Lowman, J. R. 174, 185, 203
Lund, D. 36, 56

McKee, M. G. viii, 17-34
McReynolds, P. 241
Madsen, C. H. 241
Maloney, L. J. 176, 181, 189, 204
Manderscheid, R. W. 244, 262
Marble, A. 111
Margrab, P. R. 203
Marinelli, R. P. 42, 56
Marti-Ibanez, F. 22, 34
Martorano, R. D. 227, 241
Mason, J. W. 189, 203
Massy, F. C. 245, 262
Masters, J. C. 55, 57, 227, 228, 242
Mathews, C. O. viii, 206-277
Mayer, G. 158, 164, 171
Mayers, M. G. 111
Means, R. 154, 169, 171
Meeker, B. F. 244, 262
Melamed, B. G. 151, 171
Melnick, J. 227, 241
Mersky, H. 210, 212, 221, 222
Michels, R. 67
Middleman, R. R. 67
Miller, P. M. 226, 227, 240, 241
Montgomery, D. 226, 227, 228, 241
Montgomery, P. 214, 221
Moos, R. H. 39, 41, 56, 57, 135, 147, 161, 171, 226, 228, 233, 241, 262

Morgan, E. D. 153, 156, 165, 171
Murray, H. 245, 262
Mussen, P. H. 180, 189, 203

Nietzel, M. T. 227, 241

Oberley, E. T. 36, 57
Oberley, T. D. 36, 57
Oken, D. 44, 56, 225, 241
Osmond, H. 96, 97
Ostwald, P. F. 164, 171

Patchen, M. 245, 262
Patterson, G. R. 13, 14
Peretz, D. 202, 204
Peterson, C. W. 158, 164, 171
Phillips, V. 174, 203
Pierce, W. D. 226, 241
Pinkston, S. G. 227, 241

Reese, S. L. 227, 242
Reichsman, F. 133, 147
Rice, C. E. 244, 262
Rich, A. R. 226, 227, 241
Rigler, D. 174, 175, 179, 188, 203, 204
Rimm, D. C. 55, 57, 227, 230, 241, 242
Rodgers, D. A. 222
Rogers, C. 32, 33, 34
Rollins, B. 36, 57
Romankiewicz, J. A. 163, 171
Romano, M. D. viii, 58-67
Rose, S. D. 229, 240
Rosenhan, D. L. 6, 14
Rosenthal, R. 105, 106
Rosenthal, T. L. 227, 242
Royce, W. S. 230, 242
Rustad, L. C. ix, 131-147, 231, 242

Sabshin, I. 183
Sahler, O. J. Z. 192, 202, 203, 204, 205
Sallan, S. E. 174, 203
Sand, P. L. 221
Sanders, J. B. 152, 159, 172
Sarason, I. 227, 242
Scheflen, A. E. 92, 102, 106
Scherer, S. E. 226, 227, 242
Schmitt, F. E. 151, 172
Schneider, B. 245
Schneidman, E. S. 204

Schoenberg, B. 202, 204
Schowalter, J. E. 191, 203
Schroeder, H. E. 226, 227, 241
Schroeder, O. ix, 71-80
Schwartz, B. 97
Schwartz, D. B. 177, 183, 190, 193
Selye, H. 180, 192, 198, 204
Serber, A. 227
Sewall, L. G. 244, 262
Sheposh, J. P. 174, 176, 189, 204
Shontz, F. C. 41, 47
Siegel, L. J. 151
Siegel, S. E. 175, 203
Silbergeld, S. 244, 262
Singer, P. 30, 34
Skipper, J. 133, 147
Smith, P. C. 245
Snyder, R. A. 245
Solomon, R. L. 234, 242
Soulairac, A. 221
Spear, F. G. 210, 221
Spinetta, J. J. ix, 173-205, 174, 176, 177, 179, 181, 182, 183, 188, 189, 190, 193, 196, 197, 199, 200, 204, 273
Stehbeus J. A. 189, 204
Stenger, C. ix, 3-14
Stern, G. G. 245, 262
Sternback, R. A. 209, 210, 212, 222
Stoeckle, J. 20, 21, 22, 23, 24, 34
Strauss, A. 24, 33, 34
Streltzer, J. 133, 147
Struening, E. L. 225, 240
Stuart, D. G. x, 243-262, 248, 262
Sutkin, L. C. x, 225-242
Swarner, J. 176, 189, 204
Szasz, T. S. 207, 209, 210, 222

Thom, G. 21, 34
Tigerman, S. 226, 230, 242
Toch, R. 204
Townes, B. 190, 204

Toynbee, A. 176, 204
Trickett, E. J. 226, 241
Trieschmann, R. B. 221
Tsu, V. D. 39, 57

Uustal, D. B. 153, 154, 168, 172

van Eys, J. 173, 174, 187, 199, 204
Verwoerdt, A. 18, 34
Viles, P. H. 191, 205
Vroom, V. H. 245, 262

Waechter, E. H. 205
Waitzkin, H. 20, 21, 22, 23, 24, 34
Wales, E. x, 90-106
Walsh, M. B. 156, 172
Warnes, H. 42, 57
Watzlawick, T. 17, 27, 34
Weeds, L. 111
Wehr, J. 185, 203
Weiss, L. 233, 242
White, A. G. 96
White, P. 111
Willis, C. 183
Wintrobe, M. 21, 34
Witkin, S. L. 227, 238, 242
Wittkower, E. D. 42, 57
Wold, D. 190, 204
Wolff, C. T. 189, 203
Wolpe, J. 226, 242
Woodforde, J. M. 212, 222
Wooldridge, P. J. 151, 172
Wright, B. A. 152, 161, 163, 164, 165, 167, 172
Wright, J. C. 226, 242

Yocum, B. E. x, 81-89
Yura, H. 156, 172

Zeichner, A. 226, 242
Ziegler, F. J. 222

SUBJECT INDEX

A

Activities Index, 245
Anxiety, 42, 62
Assertive behavior, 81-89
  blocks to, 83-85
  defined, 81-83
  development of, 86-87
Assertiveness
  defined, 82-83
Assertiveness training, 81-89, 225-240
  cognitive-behavioral approach, 228-240
  nurses, 225-240
  patients, 54-55, 214-217
    elderly, 229-230
Attending, 59
Audio-visual aids, 50-51, 112-127
  evaluation of, 125-126
  teacher vs. recipient centered, 116-118
  types
    films, 122-123
    filmstrips, 121-122
    minicomputers, 124-125
    slides, 121
    transparencies, 123
    videotape, 51, 124

B

Blaming the victim, 154
Body image
  dialysis patients, 132
Body language, 9, 102-105, 141
  illness behaviors, 103-105
  verbal congruence, 102-105
Burn-out, 191-192

C

Cancer, 12
  in children, 173-205
Characteristics of Treatment Environments Scale, 225-226, 244

Children
  communicating about death, 12, 174-181, 193-197
  non-verbal understanding, 181
  process over content style, 180-181, 196
  with cancer, 173-205
Chronic pain patients, 22-23, 206-221
Chronic renal failure, (*see* Hemodialysis)
Clothing
  as communication, 3, 8, 9, 246
College Characteristic Index, 245
College programs, 53, 61
Columbia University College of Physicians & Surgeons, 61
Communication
  audio-visual aids, 50-51, 112-127
  children, 173-202
  facilitating, 140-147
  involuntary nature, 4-5
  mixed messages, 25-32
  omissions, 20-25
  physician, 59-67
  process, 9
  staff, 148-172
  technical information, 13, 20-27
  twelve D's, 32-33
Compliance, 24, 137-138, 149-150, 161-165
Confidentiality, 143
Coping, staff, 138-140
  confronting, 139-140
  depersonalization, 19, 153
  detachment, 139
  labelling, 139
Coping mechanisms, 18-22, 54-55, 135-140
  dependency, 19, 136-137
  non-compliance, 137-138
  passivity, 136-137
  somatic complaints, 136

verbal abusiveness, 137
withdrawal, 19, 137
CPI-MMPI, 212, 215, 218

D

Death
  children's conceptions, 177-179
  communicating with children, 173-202
  communicating with dying patients, 12, 21-25
  communicating with families, 24-25, 175-177, 179-188, 193-197
  denial, 46, 182-184
  dialysis patients, 134
  prerequisites for communication, 175-181
Defense mechanisms, 19, 153
Denial, 19, 138
Dependency, 42-43, 133-134, 159-160
Depersonalization, 43
  in psychiatric hospitals, 6-7
Depression
  in patients, 141-142, 157-168
  staff reactions to, 157-168
Devaluation by institutions, 6
Diabetes, 109-110
  and chronic renal failure, 132
Diet
  renal, 133, 137-138
Disability
  reactions to, 41-45
Double Bind Communications, 27-31, 63-64, 133-135, 146, 219

E

Environment
  hospital, 23-24, 53-54 (see also Social ecology)
  psychiatric, 9-10
  spinal cord injury unit, 9-10, 243-262
Environmental Assessment Technique, 245
Euthanasia
  psychological, 199
Eye contact, 10, 98-100

F

Family
  communication patterns, 181-189

  coping strategies, 179-180
  divorce with ill children, 185
  stand on death, 175-177
  systems theory, 13

G

Group Atmosphere Scale, 244
Groups
  confrontation-interaction, 3, 12-13

H

Health
  defined, 71-72
Health educator, 114-116
Hemodialysis, 131-147
  home dialysis, 40-41, 133, 143
Holistic medicine, 100
Hospice, 54
Hospital environment, 5-11, 53-54

I

Informed consent, 11, 71-80, 150-152
  defined, 74-76
  experimental procedures, 75-78
  history of, 73-74
  legal requirements, 75-77

J

Justice
  defined, 72

K

Kennedy v. Parrott 1956, 76-77

L

Labelling
  as communication, 6-7
  as schizophrenic, 6-7
Learning
  teacher vs. recipient centered, 116-117
Legal issues, 11, 71-80
Limit setting, 63-64, 156
Listening, 5-7, 142, 167-169
Living will, 36

M

Medical record, 11, 107-111
Mohr v. Williams 1905, 73

Subject Index

N

Natanson v. Kline 1960, 74
Needs Press System (Murray), 245
Negative staff communications, 153-154
Non-verbal communication, xi-xii, 7-9, 25-29, 90-106
   barrier behavior, 92
   body language, 9, 102-105, 141
   clothing, 3, 8, 9, 246
   disability, 94
   eye contact, 98-100
   group norms, 90-95
   institutional, 95-97
   negative, 48-50
   sex norms, 93-94, 100-101
   space, 92-95
   touch, 100-101
Nurses Interpersonal Index, 233-238

P

Pain, 206-217
   assertiveness training, 214-217
   biofeedback, 214-217
   chronic vs. acute, 206-207
   defined, 206-207
   family therapy, 214
   group therapy, 214
   measuring, 212
   models of, 207-210
   operant conditioning, 213
Paradox
   communication, 27-31
Paralyzed Veterans of America, 263-264
   Buckeye Chapter, xi-xii, 263
Paraplegia News, 263
Patient education, 13, 20-25, 36-37, 50-53, 144-145, 163, 166-167
   materials, 51-53, 36-37
Patient rights, 36-37, 148
Patient role, 37-41
Patients
   cancer, childhood, 173-205
   chronic pain, 22-23, 206-222
   diabetes, 109-110
   dying, 12, 21-25, 30, 46, 54
   hemodialysis, 40-41, 48, 131-147
   psychiatric, 5-10, 22, 30
   spinal cord injured, 9-10, 22-30, 51-54, 72-73, 78-79, 149-171, 225-262
Physical disability
   and interpersonal space, 94
Physician communication techniques, 58-67
Prisoner of War, 10
Psychological testing, 4-5
   CPI-MMPI, 212-218
Psychology
   medical, 41
   rehabilitation, 257-261
Psychosocial programs, 257-260

R

Reflection
   as communication process, 142-143
Rehabilitation process
   staff and patient perceptions, 243-262
Rehabilitation Process Scale, 247-261
Rehabilitation team, 125-127
   communication techniques, 116-121
   environmental evaluation, 248-261
   patients as members, 114-115
Relaxation training, 55
Renal dialysis, 131-147
   coping with stress, 135-140
   home dialysis, 40-41, 133, 143
   stress for patients, 132-134
   stress for staff, 134-135
Role changes, 133, 157-159

S

Schizophrenic
   pseudo patients, 5-7
Schloendorff v. N. Y. Hospital 1914, 73-74
School
   for children with cancer, 186, 197-201
Semantics, 51-52, 66
   in medical record, 109
Sensitivity training, 12-13
Sex education, 150-151
Sex-typed communication
   non-verbal, 94
Sexual functioning, 18, 133
Siblings
   of dying children, 186-187

Simulation
  in psychiatric hospital, 5-7
Social distance
  and race, 94-95
Social ecology, 244-247
Social skills training, 55
Space
  waiting rooms, 95-96
  institutional, 95-97
  as non-verbal communication, 92-97
Spinal cord injured, 9-10, 22-30, 51-54
    72-73, 78-79, 149-171, 225-262
  demographic characteristics, 158
  family care, 54
  legal issues, 78-79
  reaction to, 158-159
  rehabilitation process, 243-262
Staff
  problem-solving, 148-172
Stress
  coping with, 135-140
  patients, 132-134
  staff, 11-14, 19, 134-135, 138-140
Systematic desensitization, 55

T
Technological Research Foundation
    (PVA), 263-265
Time
  as non-verbal communication, 49,
    97-98, 143-144
Transactional Analysis, 63

U
Unassertiveness
  situational, 83
Uniforms
  in rehabilitation setting, 246

V
Visiting hours, 10, 53-54
Vietnam veterans, 3
Volunteers, 248-249, 252, 255

W
Ward atmosphere, 230-231
Ward Assessment Scale, 244
Ward Atmosphere Scale, 225-244
Ward Evaluation Scale, 244-245
World Health Organization, 71